FART

History

Your Big Stinky Guide to the

Fascinating History of Farts

WILLIAM RICHARD

FROM TIME TO TIME A SYMBOL OF VIRILE POWER OR OF GREAT RUDENESS, NOW PRAISED, NOW EXECRATED, THE FART, ALSO CALLED METEORISM, FLATULENCE, FLATUS, OR BREEZE IS ...

INEVITABLE!

EVERYONE DOES IT, EVEN THOSE WHO DENY IT. BECAUSE FLATULENCE IS NOT OUR FAULT.

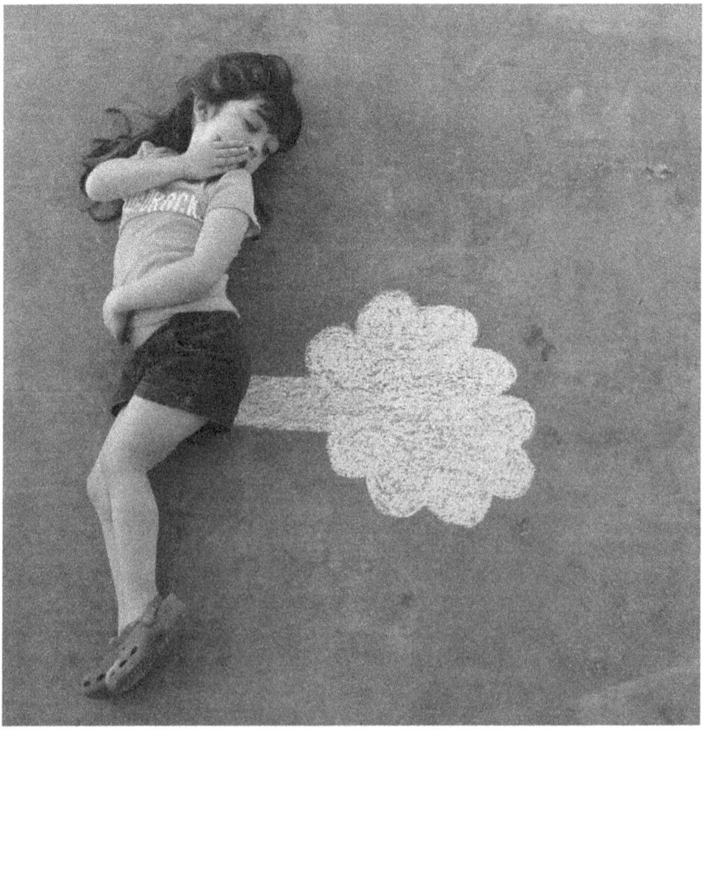

Contents

Things You (Maybe) Don't Know About Farts

Where do they start? 80-90% of the gases that cause bloating and flatulence are formed in the colon. The rest is air ingested by smoking, chewing gum, eating quickly and drinking fizzy drinks.

The causes. It was already known by the time of Hippocrates that we are all forced to free ourselves - several times a day - of the air that forms in the intestine. Responsible for this production is bacteria. There are billions of them in the colon and they are very useful: they guard the territory and prevent others - more harmful - from taking their place. They feed on any undigested food and produce important nutrients, such as vitamins K and B12. And they contribute to the formation of feces.

How they are made? The intestinal gases are above all 5 and they are odorless. So where does the stench come from? The odor, or rather the bad smell, originates from very small quantities of hydrogen sulphide (H2S), ammonia and other substances produced by particular bacterial strains.

FART History

How many do we do? On average, each individual produce from 400 to 1,200 cubic centimeters of gas per day ... equal to almost 5 glasses ... which corresponds to 12-13 "emissions".

The records of the fart. A fart is released at an average speed of 11 km / h.

Heat. Flatulence has an average temperature of about 37 ° C.

Warning: flammable gas. As most people know, flatulence can be flammable, especially when it contains large amounts of methane and hydrogen. While this may be a game for some, for others it is a problem. For example, surgeons, when they have to cauterize wounds to the intestine during abdominal surgery.

On YouTube there are hundreds of users who experience this "glowing" property of farts. Have you done it too? Well, DO NOT send us your videos.

Loud noises. The ingested air (composed mainly of oxygen, nitrogen and CO2) aggregates into large bubbles which - bursting - produce farts that are usually noisy, but odorless.

Intestinal bacteria, on the other hand, produce much smaller air bubbles, with a composition of stinking pungent gases. The result is that when the bubbles of these gases leave the body, they make less noise, but "plague" the room.

The top 10 of farting. A cow produces 300,000 to 600,000 cm3 (600 liters) of gas per day. An elephant can reach 1 million cm3 (1,000 liters), but on average it has a much lower production.

The flatulence of some animals can even be dangerous for the planet: a sheep emits 25 liters of methane alone a day; a cow reaches 280 liters. Methane is a more harmful greenhouse gas than CO2 and cattle and sheep are responsible for producing about 25% of the methane in the atmosphere. But even termites contribute: it is estimated that they emit 3.5% of the methane present in the atmosphere.

Not just beans. Some foods have the characteristic of "talking behind your back" because they contain a greater amount of indigestible carbohydrates.

The more your diet is rich in foods that contain sulfur (such as beans, cabbage, cheeses and eggs), the more unpleasant the flatulence will be.

Other times the increased frequency of farts is due to food intolerances. For example, if after drinking milk or eating ice cream you find that you are farting, it is likely that your stomach lacks lactase, an enzyme that digests the sugar contained in dairy products. Without lactase, lactose reaches the large intestine undigested, where it is attacked by hungry bacteria, happy to digest it.

A high-fiber diet also increases flatulence. But it also has important benefits: dietary fibers help control cholesterol, prevent constipation and reduce the risk of colon cancer.

They are not fatal ... You do not choke in a room full of farts.

... but dead people can "fart". The intestinal bacteria do not die immediately and continue to produce gas.

You can try to reduce flatulence with other, less drastic methods. The infusions of seeds called carminatives, that is, those capable of expelling gas from the intestinal tract, such as fennel, chamomile, anise and coriander are effective. Charcoal is another remedy. Also useful is yogurt based on Acidophilus. And finally, drugs, such as simethicone, which shatter the largest and most fragrant air bubbles into smaller bubbles.

Do Fish Have Flatulence?

Not exactly like us, but since fish also accumulate gas in their intestines, they must somehow excrete it.

Fish develop gas in the intestines and excrete it from the rectum like most animals. If we do not see lines of bubbles coming out of the back of the goldfish in the aquarium, it is because many fish "pack" their excrements (including gases) in the intestine and expel them wrapped in a sort of gelatinous membrane. These packets can sink or float, but are not often seen in the water because many fish eat them!

INFLATED FISH

The bull shark, however, uses gas expulsion as a balancing technique in the water. When it swims to the surface, it breathes air and holds it in the stomach: afterwards, it expels the amount necessary to maintain itself at a certain depth.

HERRING AND FARTS

Herring should also be added to the list of fish that make stinks. According to researchers from the Swedish University of Agricultural Sciences, in fact, the mysterious clicking sounds audible in the Stockholm bay are not produced by Russian submarines, but by the flatulence of small fish. These animals emit bubbles from the anus, producing a high-frequency sound that other herrings perceive as an invitation to aggregate to form a compact school. A strategy that allows the individual fish to decrease their chances of being attacked by a predator. According to the study, this process is voluntary: not only is the gas emitted from digestion, but the herring reaches the surface to intentionally swallow the air, which they then release rectally. An original way of exchanging information.

Farting: 7 Surprising Health Benefits You May Not Know About

Flatulence, better known as farting, is the production of a gas mixture, formed by ingested air or gases produced by symbiotic bacteria and yeasts living in the gastrointestinal tract of mammals, added to aerosolized particles of feces, which is released under pressure through the anus. It is generally associated with a characteristic sound and an unpleasant smell.

You should never fart near someone, even if it is completely natural. However, you should know that farts tell us a lot about our health and our body.

When we eat, it is normal to produce gas. It is worse to hold back than to let go. Here are 7 reasons why you should always fart.

1. Reduces the sense of swelling

If you have an upset stomach after eating, a little fart can make a big difference. It's not nice to feel bloated, especially if we can't do up our jeans. Sometimes it's the gases that inflate us.

2. It's good for the colon

We must never hold back the farts too much because it could be harmful to our health. Of course, we are not talking about holding the air in the stomach for a few seconds, but in the long run it can have negative effects if you already suffer from digestive problems, writes Woman's Health.

3. A great wake-up call

Farting is one of those bodily functions that we can never get rid of. In fact, even if they smell unpleasant, farts can predict serious health problems. If the smell is particularly unpleasant or if the farts are repeated and painful, you may need to see a doctor. Chances are you are lactose intolerant or worse, you have colon cancer.

4. The smell makes us feel good

Yes, you read that right, the smell of our farts can make us feel good. It may sound crazy, but according to some studies, farts contain gases that protect us from certain diseases.

5. Helps to have a balanced diet

We all need a balanced diet to feel good, farts tell us what foods we need to introduce. For example, if you fart very often, it means we need to eat more fiber. On the other hand, if we eat too much red meat, the farts are particularly stinky, writes Woman's Health.

6. It means our stomach is healthy

Here's a rather unusual truth: happy people fart more. In other words, it's a way to feel a little better. There are some foods that promote digestion: cauliflower, cabbage, Brussels sprouts, broccoli. Vegetables help eliminate bacteria from the stomach, and good digestion also means more gas.

7. A great relief

Nobody wants to admit it, but farting gives a great sense of relief. Why hold back? It would just make us feel bloated and uncomfortable.

Are you surprised by what you have read? Of course, we're not saying you have to let yourself go in public, but farts can be an important wake-up call for our health.

Fart Health Spies: Here's What They Reveal About Your Gut

Farting: even if at times it can be embarrassing, especially if you are not alone, in reality are a sign of healthy intestinal activity if regular, or a sign of disorders or real diseases of the digestive system if altered. Therefore, never underestimate them.

Much research has been done on flatulence, which is the production of intestinal gas commonly known as fart, sometimes referred to as a possible source of energy, especially if emitted by cows.

In 2014, a study by Exeter University even claimed that intestinal gas could be the basis of new therapies against cancer, stroke and heart attack, thanks to the hydrogen sulphide contained in them. In fact, the study was never confirmed, nor was any indication given on how to allow the acid produced by the farts to interact with the cells from the outside to provide them with the beneficial effects found.

However, science has amply demonstrated that flatulence can provide us with information on our digestive system and in particular on the intestinal tract. Here are the most common characteristics of our farts, some of which, if altered, should be communicated to the doctor as possible indicators of pathological conditions.

Frequency

A frequency of farts considered normal ranges from 14 to 23 farts per day, for a quantity of gas that can vary from half a liter to two liters per day. A very different number could reveal a pathological condition.

In fact, having the need to emit a much higher quantity of gas than normal can indicate lactose intolerance, irritable bowel syndrome, intestinal inflammation, gastroesophageal reflux, problems that cause constipation or in more rare cases gastric ulcer.

Of course, however, those who follow a diet particularly rich in fiber, such as vegetarian or vegan, will tend to produce a higher amount of gas, but in this case, unless there is really excessive production, the explanation is in the diet itself.

Smell

Farts are never scented and this is perfectly normal. Most intestinal gas is in fact odorless (hydrogen, nitrogen, oxygen, carbon dioxide, and sometimes methane), but it can happen that, due to the bacteria present in the intestine, hydrogen sulphide is produced, characterized by a decidedly unpleasant odor.

When this acid is emitted excessively, our farts manifest an unbearable odor and this too can indicate digestive problems. The compound is in fact generated by bacteria normally present in the colon, but, if this production is higher than the norm, most likely there is an intestinal problem to investigate.

Noise

Fortunately for us and our social life, farts aren't always loud (just as they aren't always smelly). The noise associated with flatulence is due to the vibrations of the gas exiting the anal canal and is strongly conditioned by the speed of expulsion (high speed, louder fart), as well as by the shape and size of the anal muscles when the gas passes.

Unlike the characteristics listed above, however, noise is not usually associated with disorders, except for problems with the anal muscle, and therefore is generally not a sign of digestive pathologies.

Eye (and nose) to the farts then.

The Pill That Makes Intestinal Gas Smell Like Pink or Chocolate

In a world still looking for miraculous pills capable of solving the most disparate health problems, here we have discovered a truly original one: the pill for those suffering from aerophagia and who want to have their own gas emissions with a rose or chocolate scent!

FART History

Yes, you got it right! It is a small preparation to be ingested able to make farts fragrant. It was invented by a 65-year-old Frenchman, Christian Poincheval, who thought people might like a range of pills that can make the unseemly and smelly intestinal gas turn into sweet and welcome emanations instead.

As the idea came to him one evening when he was in the company of friends and, due to a very abundant meal, the diners had indulged in a series of unpleasant emanations.

The new pills, all made with 100% natural ingredients such as fennel, violet, rose, seaweed and blueberries, after being approved by the health authorities, have already been sold for some years on the internet on the pilulepet.com website. According to the inventor, they could be an excellent Christmas gift and for this reason a new chocolate-scented product was launched on the occasion of the holidays.

The cost of the pills, which among other things also promise to bring benefits such as reduction of gas and bloating, is $ 9.99 for a pack of 60. And business is good, as Poincheval said: "I have all kinds of clients. Some buy them because they have problems with flatulence and others to prank their friends. Christmas always sees an increase in sales".

Meteorism: 10 Natural Remedies to Completely Eliminate a Swollen Belly

Meteorism and flatulence, what to do? Meteorism is a gastrointestinal disorder caused by the accumulation of gas in the intestine or in the stomach. Gas that is not cleared by flatulence can cause the abdomen to swell.

Speaking of flatulence, it indicates a pathological condition of formation and emission of intestinal gas due to a bacterial imbalance, with particular reference to putrefactive and fermentative germs. How to alleviate the problem thanks to natural remedies?

Herbal cure

The encyclopedia dedicated to natural health "Let's cure ourselves with medicinal herbs" (Librex, 1992) suggests resorting to herbal therapies capable of rebalancing the intestinal flora in case of flatulence. Herbs indicated as useful are green anise, star anise, fennel, dill, coriander and cumin. You can ask your trusted herbalist for advice.

Supply

Another tip concerns nutrition. Some foods may cause more fermentation and bloating than others, resulting in unwanted expulsion of gas (but necessary to clear the intestines). Depending on the individual case, the consumption of legumes, milk, meat, meat broth, sweets and sugar, leavened foods could be kept under control. As for cooking foods such as legumes, it is advisable to add a piece of kombu seaweed during preparation and to season with oregano, to avoid or limit swelling.

Chromotherapy

The same encyclopedia suggests resorting to chromotherapy, among the various possibilities offered by alternative therapies. As for the use of colors, it is recommended to perform irradiation of yellow on the solar plexus and red on the hypogastric plexus after meals, with a duration of half an hour.

Decoctions

Meteorism, increased gases inside the intestine, can be due to the malfunction of the digestive system. To bring the situation back to normal, it may be useful to resort to herbal decoctions such as mint, alchemilla, basil, hyssop and tarragon. For the methods of preparation and administration, ask the herbalist for advice.

Homeopathy

For those who prefer to rely on homeopathic treatments - always on the advice of an expert - some useful remedies can be represented by lycopodium, a particular musk, and cinchona - fundamental in homeopathy, given that the use of its peel was one of the first medicines employed by homeopaths.

Charcoal

In case of meteorism or flatulence problems it could be useful to resort to herbal remedies based on vegetable carbon. The carbon is activated according to a specific process, which allows the substance to act effectively. Among the contraindications we find laxative effects, use in pregnancy and for prolonged periods.

Essential oils

As for aromatherapy, among the essential oils recommended in case of meteorism we find essential oil of fennel, mint, sage, anise, cumin and peppermint. Herbalists and pharmacists are able to prepare remedies based on essential oils suitable for the specific case. It is not recommended to take essential oils orally without expert advice.

Lemon juice

Among grandmother's remedies for flatulence, we find lemon juice. It is believed that small amounts of lemon juice, taken with meals, can help improve digestion and, consequently, reduce the formation of intestinal gas.

Ginger

Ginger is considered a valuable aid in case of indigestion, bloating and flatulence. To alleviate the problem, you can take herbal teas prepared with fresh or dried ginger, eat a piece of fresh ginger at the end of a meal, or choose herbal remedies, such as tinctures or tablets, based on ginger.

Chamomile

Another useful remedy to facilitate normal digestion and avoid the formation of gas that will then be expelled in an annoying way, we find the simple herbal tea based on chamomile. It aids in digestion, relaxes the muscles of the intestine, deflates the abdomen and reduces inflammation. You can drink up to 3 or 4 cups a day. Chamomile teas are not recommended in case of allergy to this plant.

Swollen Belly: 10 Natural Remedies for Abdominal Bloating

Swollen belly and abdominal bloating. Here are some annoyances that could be solved by improving your eating style and trying to take care of yourself in a natural way. Remembering to chew slowly and focusing more on movement are good habits that could be part of the solution to the problem.

We indicate below some natural remedies considered useful in this regard, and we'd like to know what other beneficial solutions have been adopted by our readers to defeat abdominal swelling.

Chili pepper

Chilli, with particular reference to cayenne pepper, is considered as a suitable food to prevent abdominal swelling, as it is able to promote digestion, accelerate metabolism and the processes of absorption of nutrients, as well as the elimination of gas. and toxins. These beneficial properties are attributed to chilli due to the presence of a substance called capsaicin inside.

Fennel

Fennel and herbal tea made from fennel seeds prove to be two important allies in preventing a swollen belly. Consuming fennel and fennel herbal teas is a good habit, suitable for promoting digestion and preventing and defeating swelling. Fennel can be consumed both cooked and raw, while the herbal tea can be drunk both hot, lukewarm, or cold, transferring it to a bottle to take with you to drink throughout the day.

Apple

An apple a day keeps the doctor away, as claimed by an ancient popular saying, now considered true even by science. Enriching your diet with fruits rich in fiber such as apples allows you to promote intestinal traffic, improve digestion and prevent abdominal swelling. A real panacea for health.

Aniseed herbal tea

Aniseed herbal tea is considered an excellent natural remedy to soothe abdominal swelling due to poor digestion. Following a more abundant meal than usual, taking an anise-based herbal tea can help eliminate swelling in a short time and make digestion easier. The doses of intake and the quantity of product to be used for the preparation of aniseed herbal tea may vary according to the individual health situation. It is good to contact a herbalist.

Activated vegetable carbon

Activated vegetable charcoal is a frequently recommended natural remedy in case of persistent abdominal swelling. It can be purchased in herbal medicine or natural product stores and is usually available for sale in the form of capsules or tablets to be taken accompanied by plenty of water. In some cases, it is possible that a real treatment based on activated vegetable carbon is recommended. It is useful to consult an expert to understand if this remedy may be suitable for your situation.

Water

In some cases, abdominal swelling could be caused by water retention. It is likely that you are not drinking enough water during the day and that your body is struggling to eliminate toxins and excess fluids, which can sometimes accumulate in the abdomen. It is therefore possible to evaluate whether your daily intake of liquids, with particular reference to water, is to be considered insufficient and try to drink more, in order to understand if the swelling situation can improve in this way.

Avoid leavened foods

In some cases, apparently unjustified abdominal swelling could be due to a food intolerance. Some foods containing industrial-grade yeast could be the cause of bloating and indigestion. Through special tests it is possible to find out if abdominal swelling can be caused by an intolerance. Yeast, gluten, or dairy intolerances can have abdominal bloating among their symptoms. If in doubt, consult an expert. In general, even in the absence of intolerances, but in the presence of abdominal swelling, fried and excessively seasoned or heavy dishes should be avoided, in order not to burden digestion.

Ginger

Ginger is not only an all-round spice in the kitchen, but also a natural remedy useful not only in case of cough, cold or sore throat, but also to prevent and fight abdominal swelling. In this case it is possible to try to take herbal teas prepared using ginger root. Powdered or grated ginger can be used to season dishes such as legumes, in order to improve their digestibility.

Get moving

Abdominal bloating can be accentuated by phenomena such as poor digestion, irregular bowel functioning and a sedentary lifestyle. Digestion is improved by movement, which is considered very important for intestinal regularity, especially in the face of a particularly sedentary life. Simple walks done consistently can help. It is also possible to rely on a competent yoga teacher, who will be able to show you the best positions, suitable for alleviating the problem of abdominal swelling.

Chew slowly

We often forget about it, but the digestion of food begins in our mouth, through the contact of the food with the enzymes contained in the saliva and thanks to chewing. Chewing slowly and for a long time allows the digestion of foods to be facilitated once they pass to the stomach and through the intestines. Abdominal bloating could simply be due to rushed meals and insufficient chewing. Making an attempt to slow down and improve the way you chew certainly will not harm your health and could help solve the problem of abdominal bloating.

Inhaling the Smell of Farts Is Good for Health and Preventing Cancer

Farting is a normal part of life. In addition to sometimes causing laughter, a fart is an indicator of the health of your body's digestive system. A fart is a buildup of gas and doesn't always make a sound or leave a smell. The average person fart 14 times a day. Most will emerge without sound and are composed of carbon dioxide. When a fart leaves a strong odor, it is a sign that you have a fiber level that is healthy and there are a number of good enough bacteria in the gut.

The smell of a fart comes mainly from hydrogen sulfide.

When digesting different types of foods that have been consumed, certain types of compounds will be created. One of them is hydrogen sulfide, which creates a variety of odors that can accompany the gas out. Really bad-smelling farts are a strong indicator that everything is working fine in the stomach.

GOOD HEALTH BENEFITS

The smell of methane gas can reduce the chance of disease and help people live longer.

One such disease is dementia. Hydrogen sulfide changes the way enzymes work in disease.

If your farts smell really bad, it's not because you're unhealthy. Conversely, farts that stink mean that you have eaten types of foods that contain hydrogen sulfide. It also means that one must consume foods that are high in fiber. The only time you should worry about the smell of your fart is if you eat milk. If your milk consumption increases and significantly worsens the smell of your farts, you may suffer from lactose intolerance.

While you still need to pay attention to when and where you fart, now you don't need to fear the smell of your farts. Stinky farts indicate that your body's organs are functioning properly.

Waste of wind. Exhaust gas. Fart. There are various ways to describe the familiar sounds and smells that is released from a person's buttocks.

Why do we fart? Why the smell of farts? Talking about farts could be embarrassing and could culminate in a common point of finding out who the culprits really are. But what is certain, farting is a natural function of the living body. Everyone does it.

Here are six surprising facts about flatulence that you may not know.

Farting isn't just due to digestive issues.

FART History

A fart is a build-up of pressure within the abdomen that is released with sufficient thrust of force, which can be derived from a variety of sources. The release of air from the buttocks caused by the gas gushing into our gut from our blood, and some of the gas is the result of a chemical reaction between the bacteria that live in our gut and the rest of the food has been digested.

Different types of farts can also be caused by angioenetic edema of the intestine or as a side effect of heartburn or constipation. Some cases of wind waste, especially one that doesn't smell, is the accumulation of air we swallow while talking, yawning, chewing, or drinking.

The fart is produced by the motion of peristalsis, a series of intestinal contractions to move food waste towards the anus. This process is stimulated by the activity of eating, which makes it the reason we feel the need to defecate or fart after a meal. The motion of peristalsis creates a zone of high pressure that forces all intestinal contents, including gas, to advance towards the place where the pressure is low, that is, towards the anus. Small bubbles merge into an air bubble that is large when it heads to the "exit door".

The smell of a fart comes from sulfur and methane.

Fart gas is generally composed of 59 percent nitrogen, 21 percent hydrogen, 9 percent carbon dioxide, 7 percent methane, and 4 percent oxygen. Most stinky gases don't smell. But, some types of foods, for example foods that are high in fiber and containing sulfur (cauliflower, eggs, red meat) can produce odors. Some bacteria also produce methane or hydrogen sulfide which can add a distinctive odor. Only about 1% of farts contains hydrogen sulfide and mercaptans, which contain sulfur, and sulfur is what makes farts stink.

Farts actually smell from the start being released, but it takes a few seconds for the smell to reach a person's nostrils for you to react to the smell.

The sound of a fart varies according to the vibrations of the rectum

Contrary to the common belief that the sound of a big fart is produced by "fluttering" the two sides of the colliding buttocks, the sound of a fart is actually generated by the vibration of the rectum, or the openings of the anus.

The high-low, long-short fart sounds will depend on the tightness of the sphincter (a ring of striated muscle that surrounds the anal canal) and the pressure behind the gas that will be emitted - the combination of which causes the opening of the mouth to vibrate. Some people may voluntarily control the rate of gas by squeezing the rectum, but at night it tends to release the gas with a loud sound because the sphincter muscles are in a relaxed state.

Most people fart 10-20 times a day

In general, an individual produces about half a liter to two liters of fart gas each day, farting 10-20 times - which could fill a balloon.

Some people may fart more often than others, but not necessarily produce more gas. The problem can only be the perception of the wind is different between one person and another. In mild cases, frequency of farting is a matter of how active or sensitive the person's digestive system is, not the amount that is produced.

FART History

Often the fart is not dangerous, even if you keep it in. Often the wind blow can also indicate that the digestive system is functioning well, or vice versa, you have digestive problems, such as intolerance to dairy or gluten. But, if your exhaust is more than 50 times a day and is accompanied by other symptoms, such as severe abdominal pain, distention, or bleeding or fatty stools, contact your doctor immediately.

Fart gas is a flammable gas.

In rare cases, a buildup of flammable gas in the intestines has caused explosions during bowel surgery. Even so, it is very unlikely to be able to burn farts without the risk of injuries. In addition, fart gas has the same temperature as the body temperature, and is not so hot as to start burning.

Smelling farts is good for your health

Yes, the smell of your own farts (or anyone else's) can bring health benefits for the body. At least according to the results of the study published in the journal Medicinal Chemistry Communications. The results of the study concluded that the hydrogen sulfide gas found in rotten eggs or human gas may be a key factor in the treatment of diseases thanks to the protective function of the mitochondria.

Hydrogen sulfide gas in large doses harms the body, but this study shows that exposure at the cellular level to less of the compound can prevent mitochondrial decay.

The reason is that when the disease has forced the body's cells to work hard, the cells will draw in enzymes to generate small amounts of hydrogen sulfide to protect the mitochondria. Mitochondria essentially act as generators to release energy cells, and it acts to protect from some specific diseases, ranging from cancer, stroke, arthritis, heart attacks, and dementia.

By the way, this research is still relatively young and has not yet been tested in humans - it is still a controlled test in a laboratory against cell samples. Maybe for a while you are very grateful if there is someone near you farting.

The Hydrogen Sulfide That Generates the Bad Smell of Farts and Health Benefits

Sometimes you read news that you can hardly believe, only to discover that in reality it is scientific research that surpasses the imagination!

The smell of flatulence, normally abhorred by most, seems to have health benefits thanks to one of its essential components, hydrogen sulfide, which although responsible for the unpleasant odor, offers potential health benefits in a number of areas: from diabetes to stroke, heart attacks and dementia.

Researchers at the University of Exeter, England have designed and created the compound AP39 with hydrogen sulphide that protects the mitochondria, the "power plant" of cells, which drive energy production in blood vessel cells.

"When cells are stressed due to a disease" - explains Professor Matt Whiteman, of the University of Exeter Medical School – "they use enzymes to produce small amounts of hydrogen sulphide which is responsible for maintaining the proper functioning of mitochondria and cells. If it were not produced, the cells would die without being able to control inflammation".

The compound AP39 developed in this scientific study, exploiting this natural process, would be used to slowly transport small quantities of this gas specifically to the mitochondria.

"Our results" - explains Whiteman – "indicate that if the stressed cells are treated with AP39, the mitochondria are protected and the cells remain alive".

To clarify the extent of this gas naturally produced by the body, Dr. Mark Wood, organic chemist at the University of Exeter, adds: "Although hydrogen sulfide is well known as a foul-smelling gas from flatulence, it is naturally produced in the body and could actually be a health hero with significant implications for future therapies for a variety of diseases".

Published in April 2014 in the journal Medicinal Chemistry Communications (abstract here), the study was conducted in different disease models, delivering promising pre-clinical results. In cardiovascular disease models, for example, research shows that with the administration of the AP39 compound, more than 80 percent of the mitochondrial cell powerhouse survives in otherwise highly destructive conditions. Currently Professors Whiteman and Wood are working to advance the research to a stage where it can be tested in humans.

In the meantime, though, let's remember to thank anyone who farts in front of us, because they are doing it for our health!

FART History

Anatomy of A Brain Fart

They proved to be revolting, perplexing and infinitely amusing. Geoffrey Chaucer immortalized them in literature, Samuel Johnson defined them in his dictionary, and Benjamin Franklin urged them to be studied scientifically by the Royal Academy of Brussels.

We are talking, in all seriousness, about the omnipresent propensity of mammals to reduce the amounts of fermentable carbohydrates into what Thomas Wolfe has rightly called "fizzy and sulfuric."

We're talking, of course, about farts.

We will scrupulously avoid such unpleasant phrases as "leave a tear" or "cut the cheese". We will ruthlessly modify all colloquialisms. We are not talking about "blowing a raspberry", nor about resorting to the marginally more acceptable "breaking bad wind". We will get rid of humor from all sides and meditate only on those aspects of flatulence that directly concern the psychology of the mind. In short, we won't fart here. Our interest is far from itchy.

We will leave it to flatologists (and there are people like that in the field of medicine, poor dear ones) to delve into the issues of swelling, chemical composition, speed of expulsion and odor. Career change, anyone? It's never too late, you know. In comparison, we with an interest in psychology can breathe easily. We can, in fact, leave any further mention of guts. . . well . . . behind us, and approaching our subject somewhat safer and to the other side, so to speak.

It turns out there is a rarefied, odorless fart, we can claim as our own. It is responsible for what is known as a mismatched brain activity change. Otherwise known as - you guessed it - the brain fart. See the April 21, 2008 issue of the Proceedings of the National Academy of Sciences for the study of the University of Bergen, Norway, Tom Eichele. We are talking about serious things here.

According to the study of brain activity resulting in human error during repetitive tasks, brain farts are detectable on brain scans up to 30 seconds before an error occurs. Probably, the researchers say, brain farts are byproducts of the brain's efforts to save energy on tasks by entering a more restful state.

Normally, we only recognize a brain fart after it's a little too late. We talk out of turn or we lose our train of thought. We forget the name of someone we have known for years. We suddenly forget how to eat and raise the soup spoon too high, push it with our noses and dribble its contents onto our chins.

Of course, by "We" I don't mean "I". It never happened. Just saying.

But whatever it is, it's too late. The fart left the brain. The horse has left the barn. The cat is out of the bag. It is worth a bird in hand. . .

Uh, actually, I guess the last one doesn't quite work. Right now, I'm raising my eyebrows in surprise, shrugging apologetically and confessing embarrassedly, " Oops! Lapsus."

Why do our brains betray us in such awkward and embarrassing ways?

Probably because the routines, the bread-and-butter energy savers of our daily existence, are easy to break. Changes in context - really just simple changes in circumstances - can throw the best of us for a loop. We are often particularly prone to the disruptive influence of a change of context when we are attempting to execute a chained behavior - one in which the completion of each individual behavioral link becomes the cue to execute the next behavior in the series.

When behaviors are well established, they tend to fall into worn neural grooves. Familiarity apparently signals the brain to scale as an energy-saving measure, which leaves us vulnerable to inattention problems. We humans aren't alone in messing things up when a brain fart lets it fly.

In teaching animal homework in my previous career as a dolphin trainer, I have regularly witnessed behavior backstage which is a normal and predictable part of any learning process. Nobody learns overnight, including dolphins.

But even the fully trained dolphins who had become adept at performing all sorts of tasks occasionally had mental problems. Interestingly, dolphins react to such moments with the same surprise that we humans do to ours.

When they make a misstep during a series of routine behaviors, they often stop mid-activity, clearly aware that they have done something strange. Some of them whistle or squeak in recognition of the awkward moment. Others slap a pectoral fin against the surface of the water in mild frustration. And many of them glide below the waterline to expel a cloud of air from their blowhole in what looks, truly, like a world-class brain fart of epic proportions.

Now, isn't that a gas?

Research Reveals: Those Who Fart in F Sharp Are Smarter

FARTOWN - The sensational news coming from overseas and more precisely from the Massachusetts Institute of Fartology (MIF) has released the results of a rather singular research. The scientists' studies involved dozens of subjects of both sexes and led to the discovery that individuals with the highest IQ share a precise characteristic, namely being able to emit anal flatulence in F sharp.

The research, which lasted five years and which aggravated global warming with the accumulation of farts by 5%, revealed that this particular ability seems to be completely independent of the type of diet or age of the subject and does not even seem connected to anatomy of the anal area, as demonstrated by the 3D computer graphic reconstructions made by the researchers on direct scanning of the subjects. The ability to emit a fart in F sharp would depend solely and exclusively on the greater development of an area of the brain, located in the lower part of the right hemisphere and baptized the fart cortex. A sector of our brain that confers higher IQ and allows us to control the modulation of air through the sphincter in order to produce this particular note.

The correlation between intellect and the sound frequency of flatulences was already known in the 16th century - as it would appear from some prints recently brought to light - but today it finds unequivocal scientific confirmation.

"It was time. I've always suspected that not everyone who stinks is smart. I mean, look at Massimo Boldi. Finally, research has arrived that helps us to skim a bit: those who fart in F sharp are more intelligent. If your backside is tuned to, like, C minor, you're just pathetic farting. Eureka!" was the comment of George Van Sniffen, an anthropologist not involved in the study.

Immediately after the publication of the results of the study conducted by Dr. Harriet Stinker and her team, many wanted to know more: the curiosity to know the tone of their flatulence has become a real fever that has infected hundreds of people in a short time.

People who have started frolicking as if there was no tomorrow especially in elevators, on the sofa, in the car with the windows closed.

"Not only that - explained the local health authorities - people have begun to insert the tuning fork up their buttocks to check the correct intonation of their emissions and there have been numerous cases of hospitalizations for unnatural introductions of objects into the sphincter. And we're not finished yet! Usually, the peak is recorded at Christmas, with depression and all those tips available".

In some cases, however, there have been real dramatic situations, as happened to Brian Goodhear, a citizen of the state of Iowa with perfect pitch, stormed by a crowd seeking advice that forced him to barricade himself in home and to call the police. "Stop farting in my face" - declared the man, visibly shaken – "now my face smells unequivocally of feces, they all mistake me for Gianluca Buonanno".

Meanwhile, some Ivy League colleges have begun to select student candidates based on a record of their flatulence, replacing the classic aptitude tests. Here too, however, there is no shortage of first attempts at fraud: a nineteen-year-old from Missouri allegedly had a flute implanted in his sphincter to bypass the test and be admitted to Yale. Expelled from the University, however, he gained significant expressions of interest from the Warsaw Philharmonic Orchestra and a well-known anal sex toy company.

Joseph Pujol - "Le Pétomane"

Joseph Pujol was known by the stage name "Le Pétomane". Who among you has ever heard of this artist? Not many know his history, and a few days after his birthday it is good to refresh your memory. The life of this strange individual has been hidden for too long now; almost certainly immediately after his death in 1945 in Marseille. Let's take a step back, from the origins of the name.

Joseph Pujol was born in Marseille to a petty bourgeois family on June 1, 1857. After abandoning his studies, he began to work as a baker but something really important and unusual changed his life definitively. In fact, off the coast of Marseille, Pujol was on a boat with some friends for a peaceful trip to the sea. After a swim he noticed that the cold water was entering his body passing through the rectum. He ran ashore, and all frightened, he realizes how the water, which had previously entered, was now coming out again from his rear. He was reassured by doctors, who urged him not to worry, that everything was in order. That was the beginning of a formidable discovery for Joseph, who, intrigued and over time more and more experienced, began to practice that new skill. He was able, in fact, to suck up water or other liquids only through his anus and from the same, throw it out as if nothing had happened. Once he finished his military service, he also learned to inhale air and emit it without causing any olfactory discomfort. In short, he soon became famous on the streets of Marseille, where he enjoyed entertaining the curious and amazed people; excited enough to soon spread the word throughout the region. Ceremonies and small shows were set up where the young Pujol was able to perform more before the fateful 1887: the year in which, after a show in the city, he was so successful that he asked for more. Knowing that his skill was not an everyday thing, he moved to the capital in search of greater fortune.

The founder of the famous Moulin Rouge theater, Charles Zidler, hired this curious artist as a possible star of his shows. In the years that followed, his name spread like a gust of his air throughout Europe. The known world of the Belle Epoque was changing life, technology and modernity was the main engine for an even more advanced Western society. A different way of conceiving art was undoubtedly part of that social and cultural revolution. Joseph Pujol was so successful that he earned one of the highest salaries in the theater. His name, from that moment, was "Il Petomane", skilled in shows of "petomania".

Writers and other artists flocked to see those strange feats that the petomaniac did on stage at the Moulin Rouge almost every night. Important personalities such as Sigmund Freud, King Edward VII and the King of Belgium, Leopold II had the honor of attending one of his performances. Pujol wasn't just good at imitating animals or smoking and drinking from the rear. His evening program ranged from an accurate reinterpretation of farts in different social classes to real anal reproductions of very famous music classics such as "La Marseillaise", "O Sole Mio", "Hungarian Rhapsody" and "Au clair de la lune”. That is to say, the best of the time was reinterpreted to the sound of farts by this talented flatulent artist. The subsequent failure occurred due to his dismissal from the theater, due to continuous protests by some moralists who had gone as far as the Moulin Rouge to criticize his art, considering it demonic and vulgar.

The other reason that led him to definitively abandon the scene and the city of Paris was the outbreak of the First World War, for which he did not express much enthusiasm. We should add a nice anecdote about this too, or rather a kind of joke that makes Pujol a kind of myth. It seems that the beginning of the war was not from the killing of the Archduke of Austria-Hungary, Francesco Ferdinando, but rather Pujol himself. Hired by the French king to delight guests with a show of petomania, the Kings of England and of Prussia, Pujol thought just to honor them with their respective national anthems, playing them, of course, with a tuned farts scale. What ensued was an unprecedented din that led to war. A terrible thing, sure, but extremely exciting if it really happened; Pujol would become eternal and with him his art. Instead, he went back to work as a baker in his Marseille. Shortly before his death he opened a biscuit factory in Toulon. There are no certain sources of the exhibition at the royal palace and certainly this never happened.

To bring the name of Pujol back to its past splendor, there are two biographical films that speak of the life of this exceptional artist. In 1979 Ian MacNaughton wrote and directed a small feature film entitled "Le Pétomane". Ugo Tognazzi took on the role of the French artist a few years later with the film “Il Petomane”, directed by Pasquale Festa Campanile. As witty as they may be and quite faithful to his life, they are already old films. There is a need for fresh air for the world to rediscover the great, the unique and inimitable Joseph Pujol, the Pétomane.

True Love Begins After the First Fart

Love, real love, begins after the first fart.

You read that right ... this is a post about farts ... and about love. I repeat, it is love only after the first fart, first it is infatuation. First it is all a 'blaming' of butts to keep the breath fresh even after cracklings, a rinsing of showers to wash away the wildness, one choosing the newest socks ... so that at least they don't get pierced immediately, a trick and Moira Orfei style wig without a hanging thread. First it is a risk. The risk of dying swollen.

But one day, usually from him, the first fart escapes. Embarrassment, red cheeks, the look of a beaten dog, an apology, (then they will never say it again so remember!) And then a good laugh, together. From there it's all smooth. From there it is all relaxation. From there, finally, we women too can begin to vent our gas, always in moderation, we are ladies! But above all from there it is love!

Because it is easy to say that you love one if you see them always clean, shaved and perfumed but you want to see them at seven in the morning, with the smelly breath, bleary eyes and hair that looks like a haystack. There if you survive and you say you love him you are a gold medallist! It also applies to men!

My grandmother always told me ... "remember child, that to love each other means to share the stinks" and that's it. Except that sometimes the men exaggerate a bit!

Women Also Fart

I remember when I was 13 years old or so, I forced my father, who took me to school in the morning, to follow the boy I liked... Here, his name was Andrea and he was a year older than me. I liked him a lot and obviously I couldn't get say it. One day my father, looking for a thousand ways for me not to get hurt, told me that I had to get this boy off the pedestal. Basically, I had to downplay the idea I had of him so I wouldn't be upset if he turned me down. And to do so, he used a phrase that today, one day after my 25th birthday, I still remember. He said to me: " Alba, you have to imagine Andrea pooping, and you will see that you will like him less". At that moment, in addition to uttering a sound of disgust, I didn't think much about the scene. Back home, I thought of Andrea, the boy with that smooth and combed hair, I imagined him sitting on the toilet, busy pooping and I swear I liked him a lot less.

Now, at 25, I don't care if I picture the guy, I like pooping or farting, but, talking to some of my male friends, when it comes to a woman throwing one: O.M.G. Phrases such as "women don't fart" or "they must not fart". And then I thought, for years we women have convinced ourselves to believe that we are the wrong ones, the ones who have too many expectations from the male gender, they put you on a pedestal. Well, men, news flash, EVEN WOMEN FART; get us off that pedestal you put us on (gently for God's sake because we are always the drama queen of the situation).

FART History

Why can a man let himself go and a woman cannot? If we go for sushi and order steamed dumplings, how can we expect not to go home and spend the night farting? Do you know how bad it is to have to deprive yourself of such a natural thing? I remember once, in order not to fart, I was imploding, I was turning purple, that I felt the very air retrace the intestinal path in reverse and at moments I was having a cerebral embolism. All this for ...?

So, guys, I'll give you some advice: if it disgusts you to think that a woman can throw a harmless fart (at best it smells like a sewer), think that Beyoncé poops, that Monica Bellucci farts and smells herself and, maybe, she laughs alone because she is ashamed of the stench she made. In short, those who fart freely are happier!

The Farts Festival. In Japan: The Only Event Where You Can 'Listen, Watch and ... Smell '

An event not really for everyone. On March 3, in Japan, the festival 'Listen to all the farts of beautiful women' will be held, an appointment - explain the organizers - designed "for the 120 million lovers of farts in the world".

To report the news, in addition to the Japanese newspapers, is the Sun, which reports the words of those who created the event: " Lefkada Shinjuku is the only place in the world where you can stimulate sight and smell with beautiful women who produce various types of farts". The girls, who are porn stars, fart in skimpy clothes, in swimsuits and with different outfits.

There will also be a fart battle within the Festival.

However, there could be some unexpected events: on the description of the event, we read: "You will understand that the performances depend on the physiological state of the girls, and farts may not always succeed".

Are you curious? The ticket to participate costs 27 US dollars.

Japan: 24 Things You Don't Know Until You Go

Before going to Japan, I seemed to have studied enough about the customs and culture of the place but ... I was wrong! Once there I noticed a lot of things about Japan and the Japanese that I never imagined. Here are my thoughts, in a nutshell, on this Asian country with the funniest people you will ever meet.

Japan in pill form: everything you discover on your first trip

1) Japan is a super-male country
2) The Japanese eat a lot of eggs and yet they live 100 years ... (This story of cholesterol in the yolk cannot be right!!)
3) You can't blow your nose in public because it's rude, but you can safely fart without any problem
4) There are also fat Japanese people
5) In Japanese the word "no" is never used (practically equivalent to a go to hell...)
6) Ramen (which is considered a poor dish) is probably the dish you will miss the most
7) The green of the gardens is something indescribable
8) 1kg of tomatoes costs the same as a gold bar
9) The poor practically do not exist and therefore there is no crime
10) Onigiri are addictive
11) The Japanese are not gifted with problem solving: ask them for a minimal modification and they will die
12) Traveling in Japan is very easy even if you don't know the language
13) There are public toilets everywhere and they are all immaculate
14) In Japan you can eat very well with two lire
15) The Japanese do not give you a discount

16) You don't smoke on the street but in restaurants you do, go ahead and understand!
17) The Japanese can sleep anywhere
18) The Japanese are obsessed with packaging and use an indescribable amount of plastic (but it seems that they recycle 99 % ... at least so they say!)
19) Vegans and vegetarians don't have an easy time in Japan
20) The Japanese are always elegantly dressed
21) The Japanese are very precise but also very inefficient
22) The Japanese have drawn heavily from Chinese culture (alphabet, religion, architecture ...), let's say they invented little and nothing
23) Earthquakes and wars have destroyed practically everything, what can be seen today at most dates back to 2/3 centuries ago
24) Walking around the alleys at night in Tokyo is priceless

Japanese Burps and Farts

Didn't I have anything better to write? Ok, you are right, but I am curious about a subject that is not as stupid as it seems from the title, which is provocative.

At least we have all heard that for the Arabs the burp at the table is a sign of satisfaction with the meal, so much so that it is remembered to play down when a belch escape. It seems that in India the fart is serenely performed, as if it were a cough. A few months ago, I discovered that the Chinese spit happily on the ground and with commitment.

In Italy I have seen and heard all sorts of rudeness (insults no longer have any value for motorists), but I have never heard of someone who in public, among strangers, performed vocally or anally, as if it were a species of taboo.

However, between friends or family, it is common fact, usually men laugh and women pose as scandalized but then play the game, or actively participate.

So, I wonder how the Japanese behave:

A) they perform freely in any of the aforementioned events
B) they behave more or less like the Italians (that is, they do not dare in public, but in private the inhibitions fall)
C) always maintain decency, even among friends: certain things are never tolerated, nor do they laugh

A South African Pastor Farted on People's Faces

Hallowed be your scent

It sounds like a joke, but it's not. Apparently, there is a pastor in southern Africa who uses farts as a religious practice by farting directly in people's faces as a healing process to solve their physical and spiritual problems. Pastor Christ Penelope, of SevenFold Holy Spirit Ministries Church in Siyandani Village, Limpopo, South Africa, created a stir online for this unorthodox method after a photo of him sitting on people's faces, apparently farting on them, became viral.

However, a church attendee complained, "When we come to church it's because we need prayers, not to be farted at." However, Pastor Penelope defended her methods, insisting that she was simply demonstrating the power of God.

“Just as God put Adam into a deep sleep, it is a similar thing. God did everything with Adam's body while he was on the ground in a deep sleep. He felt nothing. The Bible says Adam complained that God hurt him,” the pastor said.

According to the pastor, farting near the person's nostrils is important for the "healing power" to enter the body to do its job.

He then added: "When they wake up from deep sleep, they will tell you that they have not heard anything. It is the power of God and those who needed healing are later healed while others arrive at that time. Remember that when people try to tarnish your image, that's where He shows His glory. As long as the souls are conquered in the kingdom, he who sits on the throne laughs at his enemies".

Surprisingly, many people even wait up to two months to meet him and get farted on, while others even collect his farts in containers.

However, other pastors disagree with Pastor Penelope's method of healing, because nowhere does God say sit on people to heal them.

Bishop Miso Mabunda of Meadowlands agrees, "These are exactly the actions the Bible has warned us against. It is said that at the end of the world there will be people who will do things that will shock us. My advice is that people follow the right path together with the Lord, because the end is near".

Pastor Penelope then reacted to the criticism and said: "I don't fart on people, I heal people."

After holy water, farts could also become a new blessing tool.

7 Farts That Changed History

A single fart that caused 10,000 deaths and the fabulous farts that made fame and money.

It may be hard to believe, but a few farts or fart stories were enough to make a big impact and make it to history.

1. The fart that started a conflict: in 44 BC 10,000 died in Jerusalem.

It is described in the bestseller, The Jewish War, that a soldier, who was opposing the Jewish people, insulted them by farting and cursing while they were having a religious ceremony. This situation offended them. So, they started throwing stones at the soldier.

When the Jews started throwing stones at the soldier, a Roman commander called for intervention to stop and attacked the Jewish people. The Jewish people trampled on themselves as they tried to escape.

2. The fart that caused a rebellion in Egypt in 569 BC

According to Herodotus, who was a Greek historian, there was a rebellion in Egypt that made Apries, the king of Egypt, worry about his power. To calm the crowd and stop the rebellion, Apries sent one of his commanders, Amasis, to suppress the rebellion. However, the rebels crowned Amasis the new king.

After this, Apries sent his popular advisor, Patarbemis, to handle the situation and talk to Amasis, but in response, Amasis farted in front of Patarbemis and told him to "take him back to Apries".

According to the Greek historian, there is no evidence as to how the message was communicated, but Apries reacted by punishing the messenger and cutting off his nose and ears. Apries' reaction was so merciless that everyone heard about it and this made the rebellion against Apries even stronger. Eventually, he secured the official reign of Amasis from 569 to 525 BC

3. Henry Ludlow's inspirational fart in Parliament in 1607.

According to Tadshistory: "Henry Ludlow was an English politician who sat in the House of Commons between 1601 and 1611".

Tadshistory explains that during a speech, "Henry let out a resounding fart. The Chamber burst into laughter. And then, the members discussed the procedural issues related to the fart incident. The incident was later described in the following popular poem":

"No such art has ever been given to tuning a fart.

FART History

Downe gravely approached Sir John Cooke and
traced her message in her book.

Fearie well, said Sir William Morris, Soe:

But Henry Ludlowes Tayle mourned Noe.

Up begins one fuller of devotion

L ' Eloquence; and said a very bad move

Not so nor did Sir Henry Jenkin say.

Movement was good; but for stincking

Well said Sir Henry Poole was a bold tricke

To Fart in the nose of the bodie pollitique

Indeed, I confess quoth Sir Edward Grevill

The question is Selfe was a bit uncivill

Thanke God quoth Sir Edward Hungerford

That this Fart did not turn out to be a Turdd "

"This poem has become one of the most popular comic political poems of the early Stuart era and has proven to inspire and become a model for a genre of political poetry, usually starting with the same ten or twelve lines"
- Source: Tadshistory

4. Flatulence humor as a scientific essay for the Royal Academy of Brussels in 1781.

When Benjamin Franklin was working in France as a US ambassador, he heard about a call for scientific papers from the Royal Academy in Brussels. In response, he wrote an essay called "Fart Proudly".

According to Wikipedia, "the essay goes on to discuss how different foods affect the smell of flatulence and proposing scientific tests on fart. Franklin distributed the essay to friends, including Joseph Priestley (a chemist famous for his work on gases)."

This was considered to be one of the funniest essays of that time. He challenged scientists to create a drug to scent farts ... Includes lines:

"A few stalks of asparagus eaten will give our urine an unpleasant smell; and a turpentine pill no bigger than a pea will give it the pleasant smell of violets. And why should it be considered more impossible in Nature to find Means to make a perfume of our wind than of our water?"

"I have reviewed your last mathematical question of the award, proposed in place of one in Natural Philosophy, for the following year ... So humbly allow me to propose one of this type for your consideration, and through you, if you approve it, for the serious investigation of learned doctors, chemists, etc. of this enlightened age."

"It is universally known that a great deal of wind is created or produced in the entrails of human creatures in the digestion of our common food. That

allowing this air to escape and mingle with the atmosphere is usually offensive to the company, with the fetid smell that accompanies it. So that all well-educated people, in order to avoid offending this offense, forcefully restrain the efforts of nature to discharge that wind".

- Source: teaching of American history

5. The farts that made fame and money in 1892.

Joseph Pujol was an extraordinary person with the special ability to inhale air through the rectum and then expel it.

He discovered his talent swimming near his home on the Cote d'Azur. According to Retro magazine, while swimming he discovered that he could "inhale" the water with his sphincter. An article in Atlas Obscura explains:

"At first Pujol used his talent to shoot in the water at incredible distances (up to five meters when he was an adult), but he soon discovered that he could get some air in too, and release it however he wanted."

After a career in the military, he began performing in music venues. With the stage name Le Petomane - " Fart maniac " - he became famous and "sang" the famous French songs, "La Marseillaise " and " Au Clair de Lune" with farts. In 1892, Joseph Pujol became famous for his "fatigability" and gave performances at the Moulin Rouge.

He could even use his farts to play the flute, blow out candles, and impress audiences with other fun farting activities.

6. The record fart.

This fart had an impact on history as it made it into the Guinness Book of Records for the longest fart ever: Bernard Clemmens' 2 Minutes 42 Seconds.

7. The legendary fart that ruined a marriage.

Although this fart and its story are just a legend, it has come down to history as one of the funniest and most read stories in A Thousand and One Nights.

"In the Middle Ages, a wealthy Yemeni merchant named Abu Hassan married one of the most beautiful women in the region and organized a lavish wedding banquet to which he invited notables from near and far."

"The groom ate and drank with gusto during the party, perhaps too heartily. When he got up from his chair to go to his bride's room, he let out a loud fart. Mortified, Abu Hassan walked away from the bridal chamber, headed for the courtyard, saddled his horse and went off into the night, weeping bitterly. It was the beginning of a strange and long journey and exile, which would have put that of the Earl of Oxford to shame."

"Disguised as a dervish, Abu Hassan wandered around his hometown for a week, eavesdropping on the possibility that he might hear any mention of his name. Finally, sitting by the door of a hut, he heard a young girl ask her

mother: "When was I born? One of my friends needs an appointment so he can cast my luck."

"The mother replied, "Darling, you were born the night Abu Hassan farted." A disappointed Abu Hassan got up and immediately fled his hometown, this time for good. As he said: "My fart is become a date - it will be remembered forever." He eventually returned to India, where he remained in self-exile for the rest of his life."

- Source: History Collection

American Students Invent the Fart Detector

Many of us, as students, spent a lot of time with peers discussing who was doing the most devastating farts. Miguel Salas and Robert Clain, students at Cornell University, decided in their last semester to do something more to resolve the debate: they invented a fart intensity detector that ranks flatulence by its overall charge.

The project, made for one of the engineering courses, was initially opposed by the professor, not because he thought it was in bad taste, but because he believed that it was not possible to find a way to measure human emissions.

In any case, the two were able to produce an instrument that classifies the gases emitted, by sound, temperature and concentration of methane, winning the highest marks and the admiration of all fans of the genre all over the world.

But to find out more about this fascinating invention, we spoke to Miguel Salas ... It took a lot of time, but not a lot of money

According to Salas, he and his partner spent more than 175 hours each on the project, but the total price, including the cost of the methane sensor donated by an admirer, was only $150.

It is easy to use

The fart detector is enclosed in a special box which is supported by a tripod which allows the instrument to be placed close to any potential "farters". It is also equipped with a fan that turns on and blows away the stench if the flatulence reaches alarming levels in the rankings.

They prepared themselves by eating cheese and beans

While Salas explains that they ate a lot of cheese to test the machine, the colleague says the beans make the loudest farts.

Caution is never too much ... the laboratory could become mephitic

Their girlfriends helped them test the machine

Although they are two aspiring electronics engineers who spend their days ruminating on the intensity of farts, the two do not disdain women at all. And the amazing thing is that women don't disdain them. In fact, their non-imaginary girls have made themselves available to test their invention. "The main difference tends to be in the sound," Salas said, explaining what changes between male and female flatulence. "Girls don't make very loud noises, but when it comes to smell there isn't much difference."

We think this would be very successful in Japan.

Salas can't see a market for this invention, but we're not so sure. Having seen videos showing Japanese games involving farting competitions and manipulations, we think that if nothing else there could be a big demand for Salas' invention in the land of the Rising Sun.

The Universe Was Born from Intestinal Gas, Here Is the New Cosmopetology of Hack

I believe that due attention has not been paid to the new proposal of scientific culture put forward by Margherita Hack when she said that she would explain the Big Bang to children as a great fart of the universe from which everything we see was born. The analogy poses a subtle epistemological problem arising from the fact that fart is contained in the intestine. Therefore, we are faced here with the paradoxical case of the container becoming contained.

The universe before the Big Bang was extremely compressed, practically point-like (almost like Euclid's point, "that which has no parts") and from this atomic entity a colossal fart exploded that included the "intestine" that had produced it. Thus, the human body is only apparently solid, in reality, it is a fart expanded by a pinched and compressed micro- intestine. After all, as Hack says, the stars are only balls of gas, or parts of a fart. Likewise, there is no reason to believe that the brain is anything other than a fart producing those little farts that are thoughts - including Hack's, it won't hurt, as she herself observes, that someone "in the stars see romance but it's all lies." In short, to paraphrase Sraffa, thought is the production of farts by means of farts.

However, another problem arises, in addition to that of the stench which, however, we leave out because it is too complex: that is, does the universe stink or not? Is it a methane-based or sulfur dioxide-based fart? Difficult to establish from the inside, you risk getting caught in some logical paradox. The problem raised by the fart theory is similar to that of the chicken and egg: what was there before the Big Bang? According to Ilya Prigogine before, there was another universe, so expanded that it collapsed at one point to give rise to a new Big Bang, so the cosmic process would be a sequence of collapses and explosions separated from the singularity points in which the Big Bang occurs. Now the vision of Hack (in honor of which we propose to call those singularity points "Hack points") allows us to concretely see the cosmic process as a sequence of farts that expand until they collapse in a point-like way to open the way to always new and immense farts.

We learn that Francis Fukuyama, (specialist in "deaths" that never happen) after the end of history has decreed the end of the human. The American essayist David Brooks, in his work, The Social Animal, has decreed the end of theology and philosophy. In turn, Stephen Hawking decrees that "philosophy is dead, we just have physics." Alexandre Koyré argued that without influential metaphysics, science is dead. Let's stop with this pessimism. There is no need to fear: we now know that science no longer really needs philosophy. From now on it will rest on the solid foundations of cosmopetology.

FART History

The Most Beautiful and Funny Phrases and The Best Aphorisms About Farts and Flatulence.

The fart, a vulgar but more common way to indicate flatulence, also called wind, gas, flatulence, or windiness, is the noisy emission of intestinal gas from the anus.

It is excess air retained by our body, the noise of which derives from the vibration of the rectum, and which is composed of 59% nitrogen, 21% hydrogen, 9% carbon dioxide, 7% of methane, and 1% of hydrogen sulphide gas. Its stench is determined by the presence of sulphides and depends on what has been eaten before; among the foods that generate more flatulence there are: beans, cabbage, eggs and cheeses. You should avoid holding them in constantly, as this could change normal bowel activity and cause severe painful cramps. Since they travel at a speed of 3 meters per second, therefore more than 10 kilometers per hour, it is assumed that it takes about 10-15 seconds before the nearest can smell them.

On this page you will find a collection of phrases, aphorisms and quotes about farts, to be dedicated to people who do not hide flatulence or to those who recently had embarrassing moments due to farts.

Sentences

Nobody is listening until someone farts. (Anonymous)

Do I mind if you smoke? Do you mind if I fart? (Anonymous)

We're here on earth to go farting around. Don't let anyone tell you anything different. (Kurt Vonnegut Jr.)

Have you heard the latest? No? It's because I did it slowly ... (Claudio Bisio)

When one laughs, he has the whole world at his feet, but if he farts, he finds himself alone. (Gordon Burley)

Do you know how to tell when a fly farts? Suddenly it flies straight ... (George Carlin)

Women and farts run away ... even if you don't them want to. (Stefano Benni)

If two people are in the elevator and one of them farts, they both know who did it. (George Carlin)

The fart is an inalienable right written in large letters on the toilet paper of human rights. (Dario Cassini)

There are days when the only moment of well-being ends up being a fart. (Jean-Marc Reiser)

Farts, let's face it, are a prominent element, especially in the lives of many males. An added value. You just enjoy. You brag. Laugh. Do the races. There is nothing that makes you laugh more than a fart breaking the sound barrier. Even that refined intellectual Dante, being male, did not resist and in Hell he put Barbariccia who made a trumpet of the ass. (Luciana Littizzetto)

FART History

Never confess a fart in public. It is an unwritten law: the most rigid of American etiquette protocols. (Paul Auster)

Let's not forget that even Romeo and Juliet occasionally farted and scratched their asses. (Charles Simic)

There is more talent in the smallest of my farts than in your whole body. (Walter Matthau)

During an interview they asked me what my worst flaw is and I replied 'flatulence'. That's why I have my own office. (Dan Thompson)

*The fart does not discourage him! (*From the movie Dumb & + Dumber 2)

Most people like to read their own writing and smell the stench of their farts. (WH Auden)

Jazz music is like a fart: only those who make it like it. (John Coltrane)

My wife farted when she was nervous. She had a number of wonderful weaknesses. She used to fart in her sleep! [laughs] Sorry if I tell you this. Once it was so loud it woke up the dog! [laughs] She woke up too and said "was it you?" and I "yes", I didn't have the courage. (From the movie Good Will Hunting)

And he made a trumpet of his ass. (Dante Alighieri)

Life is as short as a butterfly's fart. (From the movie Me, Beau Geste and the Foreign Legion)

A man who farts in bed is a man who loves life. (Muriel Barbery)

You men have a big belly too. Only you give birth in a gaseous form! (Luciana Littizzetto)

FART History

Fish are the most unfortunate beings on earth. Have you ever thought about it? A fish can't ignore it when it's farting. (Daniele Luttazzi)

Marry me and you will fart in silk sheets for the rest of your life. (Robert Mitchum)

I love the smell of morning farts! (From the movie Dodgeball)

Often ... when you cry ...

no one notices your tears ...

Often ... when you are sad ...

no one notices your unhappiness ...

Often ... when you are happy ...

no one notices your smile ...

But try farting just once ...

(Flavio Oreglio)

The dog is not an intelligent animal. Be wary of an animal that is surprised by its own farts. (Frank Skinner)

Forcibly retaining gases in the intestine produces four problems: spasms, dropsy, colic and dizziness. (Salerno Health Regulations)

What is a fart? The last breath of a bean before flying into the sky. (Anonymous)

An employer's fart is music to his employees' ears. (Mokokoma Mokhonoana)

FART History

The truth is sometimes like a fart: embarrassing and inappropriate. (Anonymous)

Why do men fart more than women? Because women don't shut up long enough to increase the pressure. (Anonymous)

- Dad, dad, dad, tell me do farts weigh?

- No, Pierino!!

- So, I shit on myself.

(Joke)

Life is like a fart, it's not the noise you make that matters, it's the trail you leave behind! (Salvatore Salvax Calabrese)

- A woman farting: embarrassing consequence of digestion, yuck.

- A man farting: fun, self-expression, a way to bond with one's fellows.

(Anonymous)

Maturity is not measured by age but by the greater or lesser ability to do silent farts. (MaxMangione, Twitter)

Finished romances are like farts: you hope to have left them behind but a memory of them always hangs in the air. (MaxMangione, Twitter)

Farts are just the ghosts of the things we eat. (TweetComici, Twitter)

A man does not write poetry. He doesn't taste silences, but he breaks them with farts. (Grim Reaper, Twitter)

In farts there is all the comedy you need. (marcosalvati, Twitter)

FART History

I'm really maturing: now when they pull my finger, I don't fart anymore. (Twitter)

A man's maturity is measured by how far he lifts his leg while farting. (robgere, Twitter)

You announce a colossal fart and then:

- It fails

- Piccinini screams NO GO!

- Disappointment in the stands

- The friend with the match goes away

(MaxMangione, Twitter)

A fart is like a kiss: it is the prelude to something bigger. (MaxMangione, Twitter)

You can have a beautiful woman, a beautiful car, but a friend's approving look for a well-done fart is unmatched. (Lux_n, Twitter)

Gasoline to go to her: 10 $

Cinema: $ 15

Romantic dinner: $ 40

Releasing that pent up fart all evening is priceless.

(estenbandeado, Twitter)

A romance can't be called intimate until she farts in front of him. (Losca71, Twitter)

That awkward moment when you make a noise that sounds like a fart, but it wasn't and then you do it several times to make it understood. (TweetComici, Twitter)

Holding back those who want to leave is like holding back a fart. It doesn't do any good, except to make you feel even worse. (Masse78, Twitter)

What then sex is nothing more than holding back a fart for half an hour. (manuela_reich, Twitter)

If your boyfriend farts and won't let you smell the stench, he doesn't really love you. (estenbandeado, Twitter)

I'm one of those romantic people who when he farts in front of a young lady says "Love is in the air". I know, few men remain like me. (estenbandeado, Twitter)

Nobody talks about the real problems in life, like when you fart at work. (Pao_LOST, Twitter)

"When I fart, he stinks."

Referring to his cabinet chief

GEORGES BENJAMIN CLEMENCEAU

"I miss your gas." VASCO MIRANDOLA

"There is more talent in the smallest of my farts than in your whole body. [Turning to Barbra Streisand]. "

WALTER MATTHAU

"Poor Ambrosini used to say that certain disputes can only be resolved with the physical act: the fart, the burp and so on." ARRIGO CAJUMI

"You can't fart without changing the balance of the universe."

PHILIP K. DICK

The Fart Through the Ages

Ever since the world had

for living Adam and Eve

it was in vogue with everyone

to cover the front,

no one ever thought, strange,

to cover the backside.

The most discreet farts

disturbed the quiet

and then the sweet sounds

did not hit the trousers

The fart of great glory

she covered herself in history

Ever since the buggers,

of very expert farts,

FART History

for excess of measure

the opening was blocked,

the Romans then subdued

they did not restrain excesses.

But Augusto Emperor

he farted at all hours

and the very perfect court

farted on the label

and even in severe cases

slaves farted

It is said that Tiberius

fart serious serious

that Caligula the tyrant

farted all year round

and more than one every morning

Catiline made it

Marco Tullio in the Campidoglio

it left them like oil

and they were certainly not few

ask the geese;

and even the Vestals

the lights were turned off

Cicero for hours

he chatted with his ass

then those of Cariolano

they could hear from afar

and with a slap on the tripe

Agrippa was also farting

Muzio Scevola and Porsenna

they brought some as a gift

at the feasts of Hymenaeus

where the consul Pompey

and even more the great Lucullus

farted for amusement

the whole of Rome farted

from morning until evening,

FART History

it farted in style

also, the female sex;

while Cincinnato instead

he made them in the middle of the meadow

Napoleon farted

even to the roar of the cannon

"The battle is not lost"

and Cambrone replied "shit",

which is the safest thing

if there is fear in between.

He farted like thunder

even Cleopatra from her throne

in contrast to Agrippina

that I did on the sly

and Cornelia to her jewels

made them burdens

He did them relentlessly

Disdainful Messalina;

FART History

he farted very happy

the sweetest Beatrice

and the great father Dante

he smelled them all

Boccaccio's farts

then they left you freezing.

Tasso also farted

imitating the double bass.

While instead Machiavelli

uprooted the saplings.

And the great poet Alfieri

filled baskets with them.

The great Volta with the Pila

he always lined up,

Paganini darkened

to make children laugh,

while instead the good Pascal

he did them on the stairs.

FART History

Of Archimedes it is usually said,

that would also obscure the sun

while with brush strokes

Raffaello made her

and the great Cimarosa

made it noisy.

After what has been said

it cannot be called a defect

if we too sometimes

we do them at full speed

therefore, it is logical and prescribed

what fart me

About Flatulence...

Commonly known as farts, when they escape, they always arouse some reaction: horror or laughter.

Having bloating or accumulation of intestinal gas is a topic that many people politely prefer to avoid dealing with others. However, the release of gas is a natural and essential process for the normal functioning of the body.

Here are 20 things you probably didn't know about flatulence

1. Definition

We speak of farting when the body accumulates intestinal gas and feels the need to expel it. This gas comes from bacteria and / or various chemical reactions that occur in the intestine as a result of the daily diet.

2. The "founder"

Benjamin Franklin is well known in American history as an inventor, publisher, writer, but most of all as one of the founding fathers of the United States and a prominent politician. What most people don't know is that he wrote a scientific essay on swelling called "Fart Proudly".

3. The speed

Many people wonder how quickly air is expelled from the body when they sneeze. And the fart? The average speed of a fart is 11km / h.

4. The fart fights

Some people have a great admiration for Japanese history, known for its elegant kimono-clad women and formidable Katana (sword) warriors. In addition to courage and elegance, the Japanese also have a keen sense of humor. Indeed, during the Edo period (1603-1868), some paintings depicted popular events including the "fight against fart" which was very popular among the Japanese.

5. Prohibition of farting

The diet of astronauts is mostly controlled by doctors or nutritionists. For example, before making their long journey, astronauts are not allowed to eat beans because intestinal gas can damage their atmosphere.

6. Not as rude as this

Some of us think farting is rude. However, flatulence can excite some fetishists.

7. The average flatulence

Well-behaved people would like to have people believe they never have problems with flatulence. This is impossible since, on average, a person expels gas at least 14 times a day.

8. Flatulence and burping

Flatulence and burping are not the same thing, the two activities consist in the emission of gas. However, flatulence contains less oxygen and more bacteria.

9. Origins

Scientists used the word flatulence inspired by the Latin word "flatus" which means "to blow".

10. The deadly animal

Contrary to popular belief, holding back farting won't kill you. However, this can cause cramps and feelings of discomfort.

"Jazz Is Like a Fart, Only Those Who Make It, Like It."

Philosophy of farting

This phrase is attributed to the American saxophonist John Coltrane and refers to all those musicians too involved in the technical and elitist aspect of music which can easily be associated with those who simply listen to the music. Too often I hear arguments from "fans" (in the negative sense of the term) coming out of the mouths of those who consider themselves passionate, and often, experts in music. It would seem that if someone listens to Vangelis' music, they cannot listen to Puccini from time to time.

FART History

Chopin would not be compatible with Metallica and the Casadei Orchestra would fight Jobim, just to name a few at random. I am the first to say that music is not all the same but the distinction I like to make is emotional. It is useless for the multi- award-winning artist with his "sought-after sounds" to present himself to me and try to convince me that the "others" only play bullshit. If my foot does not tap or my head does not sway, even slightly, with me it is in bad shape.

I add, but I don't want to rage, that often those who stand as judges of music distinguishing it (in their own way) between noble and plebeian, in their past hide moments of joyful-foolish-pure-fun. Moments that remain even if you try to deny or remove them 😉

I post a video of the artist who inspired me for this post. Coltrane is not one of the musicians I listen to most often, but my little foot (at least in this piece) is tapping happily. Obviously, I can't expect anyone reading this blog to like it too; if someone thought this even for a moment it would mean that I was unable to make my thoughts understood ... fingers crossed 🙂

Actors Who Have Farted on Set

Famous celebrities are photographed doing things ordinary people might do, such as walking their dogs, waiting for luggage, shopping or reading the news. It's a very humanizing trait, reminding us that even the most famous humans can have average human traits. In fact, some of these traits aren't always too flattering ... like farting at work!

While it may shock you, it's actually not all that uncommon for actors and actresses to pass gas on set. Some even do so during live shooting of scenes, eliciting authentic and often improvised responses from their fellow artists. Whether you do it to be funny or just because you need to, the inevitable fact is that farting is a natural bodily function that everyone from celebrities to average Joes do. Do you need more evidence? Here are some examples of famous actors and actresses who farted on set.

There is no denying that the beautiful Swedish actress Alicia Vikander is one of the most talented performers in Hollywood. She was nominated for both Golden Globes, and BAFTAs, and even took home the Oscar for Best Supporting Actress for her part in The Danish Girl. With such prestigious honors on her resume, it's safe to assume that Vikander goes all-in for every role she takes on.

In a 2016 interview with British Vogue, Vikander shed light on some of the possible repercussions of her impressive work ethic. When asked about her most awkward moment, she admitted that she once broke wind while filming a scene. 'I was going to give birth in this scene ... we went to get it, and I just went there, and I farted in the take because I pushed so hard!' While it doesn't reveal which movie it was shot in, one can imagine it must have been a traumatic experience.

THIS IS SOME SPECTRAL GAS

As one of Saturday Night Live's resident funny women, Kate McKinnon has truly made a name for herself in the comedy genre over the past five years. Her unforgettable portrayal of Hillary Clinton alongside Alec Baldwin's Donald Trump on SNL gave a jolt of much-needed relevance, which took McKinnon's career to another level and landed her roles in blockbuster comedy films. One of those comedies from 2016's all-female reboot, Ghostbusters. Even though the film failed to excel at the box office, reportedly losing $70 million for Sony, it still allowed McKinnon to humorously chew the stage with fellow SNL alumni Leslie Jones and Kristen Wiig.

It should come as no surprise that the trio, along with her friend Melissa McCarthy, brought a lot of laughs to the Ghostbusters set. In an interview with Weekly Entertainment, McKinnon got a little gassy during filming. 'Okay, whatever. I farted on camera,' she said. 'I'm starting to think that something is wrong with me ... I've never been to a gastroenterologist because it's always been normal for me, but I'm starting to feel like it's too much and I should have it checked out.' Hey, at least she admitted it! Strong and proud!

GASEOUS EXTRA

Ricky Gervais is one of the most celebrated comedians of his generation. At the age of 57, the man was awarded a Golden Globe, two Primetime Emmys, a few BAFTAs and a couple of British Comedy Awards, not to mention countless other nominations earned throughout his historic career. It's good to know that even with such a grand resume, the once 'funniest man alive' is still a childish joker behind the scenes.

During an award-winning episode of his Extras series, Gervais shared the screen with Kate Winslet. According to Winslet, Gervais did her best to make her break the wind-blowing character. 'Ricky Gervais is terrible because he tries to fuck with you,' she revealed. 'He'll fart in the middle of a scene and won't smile.' The gas must not have been that bad, because Winslet still looks back on her time on Extras with great respect. 'I don't think I've ever made it through a take without making me laugh.'

PARKS AND FLATULATION

Parks and Recreation may have experienced a shaky start, plagued with low ratings and cancellation questions, but after seven seasons and a prestigious Golden Globe Win, it's safe to say the show is a huge hit. With a cast that includes comedic geniuses like Chris Pratt, Amy Poehler, Aubrey Plaza, Aziz Ansari and Nick Offerman, how could it not be? Even years after the final episode aired, the show is still wildly popular and one of the most aired shows on Netflix.

FART History

In March of 2019, the Parks & Rec cast gathered in Hollywood for PaleyFest to celebrate the show's 10th anniversary. While answering questions, Aubrey Plaza revealed which cast member made her 'favorite' noises. 'It's so annoying because Nick and Pratt used to fart all the time ... and that would have made Amy and me mad!' It may seem odd to hear Chris Pratt, one of the People 's Sexiest Men of 2014 alive, would be so open about his flatulence, but it feels right for Andy Dwyer!

ALSO, TOM HANKS PASSES GAS

Tom Hanks, aka ' America's Dad,' is one of the most respected actors of the past 30 years. The two-time winner of the Dazzle only leads in a way that makes it nearly impossible not to love him, and for the most part, his films are very successful. One of his highest-grossing 2006 films, The da Vinci Code, grossed over $ 217 million worldwide, but the real 'Holy Grail' of that film was a pretty funny behind-the-scenes story that happened during production.

In an interview with Yahoo! Paul Bettany, who plays the film's main antagonist, shed light on what can happen if you hit Tom Hanks too hard with the camera. 'The first time I punched him - during the first scene I was on set doing The da Vinci Code - I punched him and he (Hanks) farted ... he looked at me and said: 'I just farted. Isn’t it funny?'... I loved him for that.'

A LOT OF GIANT DIMENSIONS

André the Giant, who sadly died in 1993, really lived up to his name. The French wrestler was a mountain of a man, standing 7'4' and weighing an astonishing 500 pounds. Although he was famous for his work in the ring, André also starred in some movies and television shows. Perhaps his most recognized role was that of Fezzik in the 1987 film, The Princess Bride. Starring alongside the likes of Cary Elwes, Robin Wright, and Mandy Patinkin, André told his copycats copious stories of their shared time on set, like reportedly picking up a $40,000 bar tab at his hotel.

While speaking with Sports Talk Florida in 2014, Elwes shared another story from André that certainly had fans in fits. 'My first day of work with André the Giant ... I must come back from being mostly dead ... he didn't finish his line, he just finished when he released the most amazing, gigantic, huge fart you have ever felt in your entire life. I mean a 15 second emission of gas ... the set boomed! Everyone thought it was an earthquake. Apparently, a giant-sized man has some giant-sized farts.

FARTS OF FURY

Samuel L. Jackson and Brie Larson evidently developed quite a bond during their time together on the set of various films. The duo, who first worked together on the set of Kong: Skull Island in late 2015, starred in Captain Marvel and Larson's directorial debut Unicorn Shop on Netflix. According to CheatSheet, Jackson is never too shy to criticize his relationship with the Oscar winner: 'We're good friends. We work well together ... It's fun to be in the saddle with her.'

The Flash: Batman Vs Superman

After singing along with Ariana Grande's '7 Rings' on James Cordon's Carpool Karaoke, Jackson and Larson each took turns taking a polygraph test. While you might expect these two to know everything about each other, Larson received a shocking response after asking Jackson if he had ever farted while filming a scene. 'All the time.' Digging in, Larson responded by asking if he farted while they were taking the lie detector test. Jackson said no, but the polygraph stated otherwise.

THE UNFORTUNATE SIDE EFFECT OF STRENGTHENING

It must be intimidating for an untried young actor to share a screen with one of the biggest stars in the world, especially if she's also one of the hottest actresses on the planet. Such is the conundrum that James McAvoy found himself in 2008 while filming the bullet-bending action movie Wanted. His co-star, Angelina Jolie, had just been named People Magazine's Sexiest Woman Alive in 2005, and had already taken home an Oscar for her role in the 2000 movie, Girl Interrupted. By contrast, McAvoy had only a few memorable roles to his credit at the time, including, in 2006, The Last King of Scotland, and in 2007, Atonement.

To beef up and look the part of an action hero, Wanted producers made McAvoy take muscle gain supplements. According to Cosmopolitan, the supplements had a pretty nasty downside. 'To be honest, it really helped me, but it came with a huge side effect of me farting violently ... It was so thick and so vigorous that I couldn't stop. When I was shooting, I was by far the biggest farter in Hollywood. That's probably not the impression you want to make when shooting intimate scenes with one of the sexiest women alive.'

FARTIN FORTE

Kristen Schaal, the side splitting Emmy nominee voicing Louise Belcher in Bob's Burgers, is no stranger to funny business. With a resumè chock full of small roles in some of the most important shows in the world, including 30 Rock, The Simpsons, Archer, and Bojack Horseman, Schaal has really made a name for herself in Hollywood over the past decade. In Fox's The Last Man On Earth, she and fellow comedian Will Forte play two of the last humans in a post-apocalyptic world. Hilarity naturally follows.

It's not hard to imagine that if you are two of the last people on Earth, you might be inclined to ... get familiar. While on the page, a sex scene between the two characters seemed logical, what happened during filming was anything but. On Late Night with Seth Meyers, Schaal admitted that the whole moment - along with a scene requiring her to eat a copious amount of beans - had an unplanned outcome. 'Carol (Schaal's character) is talking aggressively and sexually with Phil - that's a lot of diaphragm work, which is also in the danger zone of where the beans are ... I finally just looked at Will and I was like, 'I'll fart on you.' And I did. Showing no shame, Schaal proudly backed up her smelly action: 'If you fart on your scene partner it's the most intimate you can get.'

A MOTION CAPTURE EXPERIENCE TO REMEMBER

Before becoming a teenage heartthrob for his portrayal of Peeta Mellark in the Hunger Games series, Josh Hutcherson was just a talented young actor who played any small role he could get his hands on. In 2004, he picked up a small part in Robert Zemeckis' imaginative Christmas movie Polar Express, starring Tom Hanks. Via motion capture, Hutcherson played the role of a young boy who was struggling to regain his faith in Santa Claus.

Hanks played a number of parts in the film, including that of a tramp. At one point in the film, Hutcherson's character skis on top of the train with the hobo, which means that Hutcherson, fully dressed in the necessary top hat, sat on Hanks's lap to shoot the scene. In late 2017, over a decade after the film's release, Hutcherson was on The Late Late Show with James Corden, sharing a behind-the-scenes bit of the production that no one knew about. 'I farted in the scene ... That was my first big movie ... and I was working with Robert Zemeckis and Tom Hanks ... and I just farted in his face!' Although Hanks is apparently playful about it, you have to imagine that farting on Forrest Gump was traumatizing enough for a nine-year-old.

'HAVE YOU DISCOURAGED, RAY?'

Rain Man, in 1988, cleaned up at the Oscars, taking home four awards including one for best picture. For his portrayal of Raymond Babbitt, the autistic brother of Tom Cruise's Charlie, Dustin Hoffman took home the best actor for a starring role, his second time winning the award. While you might think that the actors on the set of such a high-profile film were entirely professional and formal with the camera, there is a story that provides evidence to the contrary.

In an interview with Squire, Dustin Hoffman shared his thoughts on why Rain Man was such a hit, using one particular scene as an example. 'You take away the laughs of Rain Man and it's not the same movie. When we are in the phone booth and fart, it was a fart. It wasn't written in the script. We were waiting to shoot and (director) Barry Levinson had earphones. The door closed and I let one out. We were tight in there, you know. And Cruise looked at me and said, 'Did you fart?' And I said, 'Yes'. But I stayed in character. ' Fart.' Barry heard it and came running hysterically and said, 'It's in the scene. Put it where you want.' He's a good director: someone who takes advantage of accidents. It's not often that an actor sees a toot in the camera as such a skillful moment, but it undeniably worked well enough for Hoffman and Rain Man.

The Fart Gains in Social Credibility

The green light for farts was given by a well-known fashion house, with some television advertising that made the act of farting spectacular. This was a decisive symbolic gesture: now pride took over from shame. Meanwhile, from France the news of a tablet that gives the fart a mint smell

The fashion house Dolce & Gabbana took care of rehabilitating the ethical and social value of the fart. It did so with a recent TV commercial that will certainly not have escaped the morbid or passive viewer. The spot features a young couple. The man gives the woman a watch, satisfied with the gallant gesture; this does not control the unexpected release of a light and caressing fart. It happens. At this point, the embarrassment could jeopardize the woman's demeanor, but here is the young man, who in turn abandons himself to the impulses of nature, thundering in a much more powerful way. It is the chivalrous fart, which marks the entry of today's man into the new frontier of good taste.

The fart is the inner voice of each individual. That's right, it is born within each of us - no one is excluded - and tends to come out sometimes boldly, sometimes with some hesitation due to an innate or acquired shyness. Depending on the case, from twelve to fourteen interior voices can be released per day. We are prodigious in this: we are an authentic miracle of nature. And there is little to be ashamed of, because in ancient Egypt the

Fart was even considered a deity. It was depicted unequivocally, in the form of a child squatting. And the fart was.

How? Do we all emit more or less polluted air? How is it possible? It is possible. Even the kindest and most graceful people in this world, even the most refined and noble of mind, allow themselves the luxury of farting. In short, the fart is looming, one does about it every two hours, for a volumetric total that can vary from person to person, from 200 to 2000 milliliters a day. It is the reality of the facts. Therefore, it is appropriate to say 'Health!'

The right and politically correct word? Flatulence. Yes, because every fart is flatus, puff; while for the English it is fart, and the intestinal gas consequently escapes fearlessly from the rectum, it can even be visualized radiographically. The sphincter opens and away, the concert begins. Are anti-pollution measures envisaged? Yes, someone tries.

A tiny tablet to make the fart perfumed. Yes, anti-pollution measures are foreseen, the imagination is certainly not lacking. The application of a rectal tube to avoid poisoning the surrounding environment is impractical and too old-fashioned. Can you imagine the petomaniac with an exhaust pipe applied behind? It's funny. France, which is an evolved and odor-sensitive country, has identified an easy-to-approach solution. The inventor is Christian Poincheval. He found a way to make a pill that breaks down the fart stench. From December it is possible (at least in France) to buy a pack of tablets that give a pleasant smell to the farts. With the modest sum of $6 you can choose between mint or tarragon flavor. What happens next? The tablet dissolves in the intestine and counteracts the fermentation. In short, when you are committed, the solutions are found. On the other hand, Monsieur Poincheval is not lacking in ideas. To his credit there is another invention: toilet paper decorated with comic strips. In this way, at least, while waiting you avoid carrying newspapers or books, which are too bulky. But how is it done? Does everyone sit down with their own toilet paper? Of course, otherwise you lose the thread (of the story, of course).

The composition of a fart? It is a gas charge of different concentration. There is nitrogen, carbon dioxide, hydrogen and methane largely, but not only. In general, odorless or almost odorless gases prevail, then instead, when something is wrong with the digestive mechanism, when intestinal microbes indulge themselves and gas containing sulfur takes over, then here is the unmistakable stench of rotten eggs (when it goes well). Who knows what writer James Joyce recognized in his wife Nora's farts? In a letter to his beloved, he wrote: "I think, Nora, that I would recognize your farts anywhere. I bet I'd even recognize them in a room full of farting women. They make a girlish noise, not like some fat wives I imagine farting wet and windy. Yours are sudden, dry and dirty like a witty girl would do them, for fun, at night, in a dormitory. I really hope that my Nora wants to put them on my face, so that I can smell them too".

Scientists Develop Recipe for Artificial Farts

Farts can be downright embarrassing, and many dreams of systems that effectively neutralize them. But in order to design such products, you first need to develop realistic artificial farts to test them with. Fortunately, a group of Danish scientists seem to have found the solution. They put together common strains of different species of bacteria in the lab to develop a "recipe" that produces a realistic smell of farts.

Congratulations to these researchers because the study must not have been pleasant. At first, anaerobic bacteria representing a broad spectrum were selected from an international collection of recognized cultures and then incubated in an anaerobic vessel. After 24 hours the lid was removed and the odor was evaluated by a clinical microbiology specialist.

In total, seven different combinations of two or three strains were tested. In the end, the combination of Bacteroides fragilis ATCC 25285, Clostridium difficile ATCC 700057 and Fusobacterium necrophorum ATCC 25286 was chosen as it had an appropriate smell, thus allowing the production of artificial flatus from volatile bacterial compounds. The method is easy and inexpensive and can thus aid further research on measures to neutralize intestinal gas emissions.

FART History

Science and Chemistry, Let's Talk About Serious Things

The term flatulence describes a condition characterized by an excessive synthesis of gases in the gastrointestinal tract, accompanied by an abnormal emission of the same gases from the rectum.

The causes at the origin of the phenomenon can be many. Flatulence is often caused by an increase in fermentation or putrefactive processes, resulting from qualitative and quantitative food errors. Other times it is the fault of drugs, stress and excessive tension.

Flatulence, Stomach pain

Although intestinal fermentation is an absolutely physiological phenomenon, the excessive production of gas that characterizes flatulence is often accompanied by an annoying or painful abdominal distension (meteorism), especially when, for physiological or social reasons, such gases cannot be vented.

FUN FACT: the noise commonly associated with flatulence is caused by the vibration of the anal opening.

Some people are able to control the sphincter that normally closes this orifice and, by reducing abdominal pressure, draw air into the rectum through the anus. This is the case of the famous Joseph Pujol who, more than a century ago, animated the nightlife of the Parisian Belle Epoque with a musical show based on farting. This peculiar ability earned him the nickname of "the Petomane".

Causes

Flatulence recognizes several possible causative agents. Below is a list of the main ones.

Aerophagia: excessive swallowing of air, usually followed by noisy belching. It can have a pathological basis (gastroesophageal reflux, hiatal hernia, angina pectoris, dyspepsia, peptic ulcer) or behavioral (smoking and bad dietary habits, such as hasty ingestion of food or drinks, especially carbonated drinks).

Excessive bacterial fermentation: in these cases, flatulence is linked to the ingestion of foods rich in oligosaccharides which, not being completely digested, arrive in the colon, where they constitute the energy substrate of the local microflora. These microorganisms synthesize gaseous waste products, mainly composed of: hydrogen, oxygen, carbon dioxide, methane, nitrogen and the foul-smelling skatole, sulfur, indole and butyric acid. Excess bran can also cause flatulence and abdominal tension.

If flatulence is not associated with pathology or frequent belching, it is most likely due to excessive bacterial fermentation. In these cases, we speak of pure hyperflatulence.

Pathologies: gastritis, peptic ulcer (gastric or duodenal), hiatal hernia, colitis, irritable bowel syndrome, bacterial contamination syndrome of the small intestine and food allergies, but also emotional and mental disorders (anxiety, depression and stress excessive).

How to recognize flatulence

As anticipated, flatulence is generally linked to the composition of the diet, more rarely it is accompanied by important pathologies. For this reason, diagnostic investigations are generally useless and the problem vanishes with simple dietary therapy.

When flatulence creates significant discomfort in the social context or severe pain caused by excessive gas accumulation, an accurate diagnostic investigation can still be useful.

First of all, a thorough medical history of the patient is necessary, for example investigating whether flatulence:

- it is associated with the consumption of particular foods or with certain psychological conditions
- it is accompanied by other symptoms such as changes in the hive (constipation, diarrhea), abdominal pain or faecal discharge of mucus and blood
- it is associated with the intake of particular drugs, with diseases in progress or if there is a familiarity for certain pathologies

Thanks to an accurate medical history of the patient, the doctor can at this point hypothesize the origin of flatulence, for example:

- if it is associated with the consumption of particular foods → possible food intolerance
- if it is associated with particular eating habits (abuse of sugary drinks, sweets, starchy foods, diet low in fruit and

vegetables, overeating, sedentary lifestyle) → possible loss of the optimal absorption capacity of the intestinal mucosa (dripping bowel syndrome or hyper- intestinal permeability)

- if it is associated with alterations of the hive and states of nervousness, anxiety, stress, depression, hypochondria → possible irritable bowel syndrome
- if it is associated with fever, diarrheal discharges, severe abdominal pain → possible intestinal infection in progress
- if it is associated with diseases with an important autoimmune component (e.g. psoriasis, arthritis), blood in the stool, abundant presence of mucus in the excrement, periods of constipation and others of diarrhea, with alternation of remissions and relapses → possible presence of an inflammatory bowel disease
- if associated with ribbon-like stools, age >50 years, abdominal pain, anemia and blood in stool → possible colon cancer (malignant or benign)

To confirm or deny these hypotheses, the doctor can subject the patient to one or more diagnostic tests

The traditional examination consists of collecting the gas expelled through a rectal tube inserted into the anus and connected to a syringe. The chemical analysis of these gases will therefore be able to establish the origin of flatulence: if the majority constituent is nitrogen at the base of the disorder, there is most likely aerophagia; if, on the other hand, the fart is rich in hydrogen and carbon dioxide it is a malabsorption of carbohydrates, with consequent bacterial hyperfermentation, as happens in lactose intolerant subjects. In any case, to be able to speak of flatulence, the number of daily expulsions must be greater than 25; the gas emitted must also exceed 100 ml / h. On the other hand, 10-20 passings per day are completely normal, for a total volume of about one liter of air (Bibliography: Outpatient colon proctology - treated for surgeons, gastroenterologists and practitioners, page 97).

When the doctor supposes that the origin of flatulence is linked to a food intolerance, to a bacterial contamination syndrome of the small intestine or to intestinal malabsorption problems, he can perform the so-called breath tests, certainly more practical and used than the previous test. To learn more about the topic, we suggest reading the articles on the Breath test for the diagnosis of lactose intolerance and on the sorbitol Breath test.

Alternatively, or together with breath tests, the doctor may prescribe stool tests (e.g. measurement of fecal pH) and blood tests (e.g. search for specific antibodies, for celiac disease)

When symptoms indicate a possible severe pathology, X-ray examinations of the gastrointestinal tract and possibly endoscopic examination (gastroscopy and / or colonoscopy) with biopsy are indicated.

It often happens that the patient attributes the origin of abdominal pain to flatulence, when in reality there is only an increased sensitivity of the colic wall (irritable bowel syndrome) at the basis of the disorder. Thus, one gets the impression that some foods cause bloating but, in fact, they stimulate not so much flatulence, but a series of involuntary intestinal contractions, which are perceived as an annoying sense of gaseous distension.

Intestinal Gas

Intestinal gases are 99% made up of nitrogen, oxygen, carbon dioxide, hydrogen and methane. However, the bad odor is not conferred by these major components, but by the very small percentage of sulfur dioxide, hydrogen sulphide, indole, volatile fatty acids and skatole.

In physiological conditions the quantity of gas in the intestinal lumen is quite stable, oscillating around 200 ml, with an average elimination ranging from 400 to 1600 ml per day; the composition of the gases is also quite variable, but nitrogen remains the main component. Collecting and analyzing the expelled gas can help to establish the origin of flatulence: if the major constituent is nitrogen at the base of the disorder, there is most likely aerophagia; if, on the other hand, the fart is rich in hydrogen and carbon dioxide, it is presumably a malabsorption of carbohydrates, with consequent bacterial hyperfermentation.

Causes - Why are they formed?

The predominant contribution is given by the air ingested during swallowing. For this reason, people who drink and eat hastily, or talk a lot during meals, are more prone to flatulence problems. The same goes for smokers and for those who frequently chew gum or tobacco; finally, a significant contribution to the formation of intestinal gas is given by the air contained in food; for example, smoothies and carbonated drinks are rich in it, while some antacids, such as sodium bicarbonate, produce significant quantities of carbon dioxide in the stomach. For the same reason, large volumes of carbon dioxide are continuously formed due to the neutralization of gastric acids by pancreatic and biliary bicarbonates. Fortunately, the several liters of CO2 developed by these reactions quickly pass into the bloodstream to be eliminated by breathing. At the level of the colon, another physiologically important contribution is that of carbon dioxide which passes from the blood to the intestinal lumen, crossing the mucosa; this passage is in any case bidirectional and as such also allows the reabsorption of enteric CO2, favored by a partial pressure higher than the plasma one.

As most people know, the origin of intestinal gas can also be traced back to the activity of bacteria present in the large intestine. These microorganisms ferment undigested or unabsorbed food residues, drawing energy and releasing gas; it follows that the greater the concentration of unabsorbed substances at colic level, the greater the production of intestinal gas. In lactose intolerant people, for example, the inability to digest this sugar leads to the formation of large quantities of intestinal gas by the local microflora. Similarly, the flatulence associated with the consumption of legumes is linked to their content in non-digestible oligosaccharides (stachyose and raffinose), which in the large intestine give rise to massive fermentation by bacteria.

Flatulence and meteorism

For meteorism we mean an excess of gas in the intestinal lumen, the direct consequence of which, that is, an abnormal emission of gas from the rectum, is called flatulence. It must be said, however, that several patients who suffer from meteorism (distension and abdominal cramps), have a normal intestinal gaseous content. In these cases, at the origin of the problem there is very often an altered intestinal motility, which produces rapid movements of gas with acute and painful distension of some loops.

On average, the number of daily expulsions of intestinal gas through the rectum is equal to 14 acts, while we talk about flatulence when this number exceeds 25 episodes.

Foods that increase intestinal gas

There is a long list of foods traditionally believed to be responsible for increasing intestinal gas. These include:

Beans, foods high in lactose, lentils, broad beans, peas, chickpeas, soy, simple sugars (especially fructose), polyols (sorbitol), fresh bread, turnips, celery, radishes, horseradish, yeast, cabbage, Brussels sprouts, cauliflower, carbonated water and soft drinks, sparkling wines, sauerkraut, cabbage, savoy cabbage, cucumbers, shallots, peppers, celery, onions, garlic, chilli, watermelon, melon, apple, avocado, chestnuts, walnuts, hazelnuts, almonds, dried figs and dried fruit, whipped cream, mayonnaise, milkshakes.

Much depends, however, on individual variability, in the sense that products that are well tolerated by some could be problematic for others, and vice versa. Other important factors to consider are:

- the amount of food consumed;

- the association with other foods within the same meal (evaluate both the type of foods and the overall volume of food ingested; for example, meals that are too abundant or eaten too close to previous meals tend to increase the formation of intestinal gas);
- any basic ailments (gastritis, ulcers, intolerances, etc.)
- the speed of chewing (a meal eaten in a hurry creates greater digestive disorders)
- the level of stress (intestinal disorders tend to grow as stress increases).

Cures and Remedies for Flatulence

Flatulence therapy is based on eliminating the causes that generated it.

Natural remedies

In phytotherapy, carminative medicinal plants are used, capable of preventing the formation of gas in the intestinal tract or favoring its expulsion. Among all, the best known is fennel, very useful for moderating fermentation and promoting the elimination of excess gas. Cumin, anise, chamomile, mint, lemon balm and angelica are also typical plant drugs with carminative action.

Apple cider vinegar, thanks to its ability to restore intestinal acidity, prevents the growth of putrefactive bacteria that alter the slightly acidic pH in the intestine. Its action is particularly useful when flatulence is linked to an excessively high protein diet.

Chewing and other Remedies

To combat aerophagia it is necessary to re-evaluate the role of good chewing and the need to eat meals in a relaxed and comfortable environment. Chewing enough and allowing the right time for digestion is therefore a basic requirement to facilitate digestive processes.

If flatulence is associated with meteorism, taking antacids thirty minutes after meals may be useful. The efficacy of activated carbon and other drugs with adsorbing properties is controversial.

Recently, alpha-galactosidase-based supplements have also been put on the market, useful for counteracting the formation of intestinal gas from non-digestible oligosaccharides.

Diet

In most cases, the most effective therapy is dietary therapy. The typical diet involves the reduction of legumes, cabbage, flour and all other foods that facilitate the formation of gas, in favor of others that favor its absorption. More generally, in case of flatulence it is useful to eliminate foods commonly associated with food intolerances such as milk and foods rich in gluten or fructose. Also beware of dietary products containing polyols such as sorbitol.

An often-overlooked aspect concerns the variety and balance of nutrition. The diet is in fact important to keep the bacterial flora in optimal conditions; if it is too rich in certain foods and poor in others, the risk of creating changes in the microbial populations, with consequent meteorism and flatulence, is quite high.

Drugs and Digestive Enzymes

In persistent cases, intestinal antibiotic therapy (indicated in case of bacterial contamination of the small intestine) and supplementation with digestive enzymes (indicated in the presence of pancreatic problems) can be used. The use of probiotic foods instead has the purpose of rebalancing and strengthening the bacterial flora of the colon. Before taking these products, however, it is advisable to consult a doctor.

Lactic ferments, for example, could complicate the bacterial contamination syndrome and therefore have an effect opposite to what was hoped for. These products could in fact further enhance the bacterial flora of the colon, favoring its ascent into the small intestine and causing symptoms such as bloating, flatulence, diarrhea and constipation.

Nutrition and Health. Scientific Answers to Frequently Asked Questions

No food is excluded; foods that naturally contain gas or that produce it should be eaten in moderation. Even the adoption of " correct" behavior helps to combat meteorism

Beware of highly fermented foods.

No food is excluded; foods that naturally contain gas or that produce it should be eaten in moderation. The adoption of 'correct' behaviors also helps to combat meteorism.

It cannot be defined as a worrying disorder, but widespread and annoying. It is meteorism - that is, the excessive production of abdominal gas - which periodically with spasms, distension and abdominal pain afflicts approximately 15% of the population. It is usually caused by bad eating habits - meals eaten too quickly, chewing gum chewed for a long time with the consequent introduction into the stomach of excess air, smoking - or foods that in the fermentation process produce gas or that already naturally contain, such as fruit or fizzy drinks. Often a correction of the diet is sufficient to reduce the frequency of the disorder and the manifestation of the episodes or, at best, to prevent its occurrence.

CAUSES

It is the hyperproduction of oxygen, nitrogen, carbon dioxide, methane, hydrogen gas that derives from the fermentation activity of intestinal bacteria on nutrients (especially carbohydrates and proteins, the so-called SIBO Small Intestinal Bacterial Overgrow or Bacterial Contamination Syndrome of the Intestine) or the difficulty in eliminating them, to be responsible for the meteoric syndrome. Swelling, a sense of fullness and abdominal pain appear in a temporary or chronic manner, which may also be accompanied by perceptible intestinal noises or belching. In some cases, however, meteorism can be a sign of the presence of other gastro-intestinal problems: irritable bowel syndrome, dyspepsia (digestive disorders), constipation or be related to psychological factors such as anxiety, depression and insomnia. Food choices, experts say, have an important impact on the production of gas in the intestine, but they also recommend not excluding nutritional foods that are precious only for their meteoric power, limiting their intake to small or moderate quantities. Here is what to favor or exclude from the diet against excess gas:

FOODS TO CONSUME WITH MODERATION

Milk and fresh dairy products, brassicas (turnips, savoy cabbage, cauliflower and cabbage), onions, thistles, legumes (chickpeas, beans, lentils), foods rich in fat, carbonated water and soft drinks, sparkling wines, whipped cream, frappé, mayonnaise, bread, sweets, chewing gum, sweets, chestnuts, foods sweetened with sugar alcohols (sorbitol, mannitol). Avoid drinking through a straw which leads to ingesting 'useless' air.

FOOD WITHOUT LIMITATIONS

Meat, fish, poultry, eggs, aged cheeses, vegetables (except those mentioned), cereals (excluding fresh bread). Among the fruit, prefer melon, pears, apples, citrus fruits, pineapple. Effective against meteorism are, at the end of the meal, carminative herbal teas (with fennel seeds, dill, cumin, etc ...). Do not abolish fibers, but insert them in the diet very gradually and according to individual tolerability. Under medical prescription, some preparations, available on the market, containing the enzyme alpha-galactosidase capable of degrading some components of legumes, fruit, vegetables and cereals that fermenting can contribute to meteorism can be added to dietary and behavioral recommendations.

BEHAVIORAL ADVICE

No less important, to combat meteorism, is the adoption of certain behaviors linked to a correct lifestyle and 'bon ton'.

- Abolish or drastically reduce smoking
- Do not go to bed immediately after meals
- Chew slowly with your mouth closed
- Do not speak while putting food in your mouth or chewing
- Avoid stress
- Perform regular physical activity, including brisk walking
- Check the efficiency of dental prostheses

Farty Animals

Birds and sloths don't do it, for other animals they are the only surprising possibility of salvation, says a new book

Flatulence is not just the prerogative of humans; many animals get rid of accumulated gases in the same way and - for some of them - it can be a matter of life or death. The Cyprinodon atrorus, for example, is a small fish typical of Mexico that lives in stagnant, shallow waters, hiding from predators under rocks. It feeds mainly on algae, which however in summer emit gas bubbles which are swallowed by Cyprinodon atrorus, causing it to swell the viscera. The small air chamber that forms inside pushes the fish afloat, making it easy prey. In some cases, moreover, the accumulation of gas is such as to be lethal, because it compresses the organs until they collapse. Fortunately for Cyprinodon atrorus, in most cases some flatulence is enough to get rid of the excess air and avoid having a bad end.

The science of flatulence is not yet clear in all its aspects, but it has nevertheless led over the years to research both on humans and on other animals. In our case, the accumulation of gas in the digestive system is due to the air we ingest and the fermentation of food, a fundamental process for assimilating nutrients. Gases also help facilitate bowel movements, as long as they are regularly vented outside. In addition to the most - er - sound cases, we often release part of the intestinal gas without realizing it throughout the day.

FART History

Intrigued by how flatulence works in the animal kingdom, Dani Rabaiotti, a zoologist at University College London, did some research and wrote an illustrated book on the subject: Does it Fart? The Definitive Field Guide to Animal Flatulence. As Rabaiotti told us, the idea for the book was born a few years ago, when her brother asked her if snakes also produced flatulence. He had no idea and so he got help on Twitter from a friend of his, a herpetologist, that is, a specialist in the study of reptiles. The answer was yes and also led to the birth of the hashtag #DoesItFart, which at the beginning of 2017 collected some success online, even of a scientific nature.

Put in contact through the hashtag, researchers and experts put together a shared document online where everyone could add news on the flatulence of particular animals, provided they cite precisely the sources and the scientific literature on the matter. Together with Nicholas Caruso, Rabaiotti later turned this collective work into a book, thinking it might be fun to add some humorous illustrations. The book, which can be purchased on Amazon in English, includes about 80 animal species with information and curiosities on how to get rid of excess gas.

Rabaiotti explained that flatulence in many animals is primarily due to the air they swallow while eating or performing other activities. Several species suck air into the anus, as well as expel it, for example to use it to propel themselves into the water faster or to aid breathing, as is the case with some turtles.

While working on the book, the authors also stumbled upon research explaining particular ways scientists use to measure flatulence in animals. In the case of dogs, for example: "They have developed a kind of coat with a test tube attached to the bottom. It was made for the dog to wear, with the test tube that remained placed where you imagine, leaving the dog the opportunity to walk, eat and do the rest without more invasive solutions to extract the gases ". Many other tests were performed in less creative ways, by placing animals in special rooms and detecting changes in the composition of the air with sensors. The problem is that in this way it became more difficult to understand from which orifice the flatulence came out, in the case of particular animal species.

After extensive research, the authors found confirmation that sloths do not produce flatulence: the accumulation of gas for them can be lethal. Not even birds let themselves go. The authors are now thinking of a second volume because, they admit, the book is very biased towards mammals, aided by the fact that most of the researchers who contributed to the original document mostly deal with these animals. The hope is that by involving entomologists and researchers in other fields we can discover and divulge something more, without giving ourselves too many airs.

There Is an Animal That Communicates Through Farts

Herring have an unusual way of communicating: farts. It has long been known that these fish make unusual sounds, but it was only recently that researchers realized that herring makes these sounds... with the anus.

The discovery was made only when researchers caught wild herring and then kept them in captivity to observe them, realizing that they use farts to communicate with other fish.

The fact that it is a means of communication is a conclusion the researchers came to after noting that the fish tended to fart much more in the presence of other fish, and that the number of farts was independent of the type of feeding of the fish.

While the exact meaning of the emissions is still a mystery, it can be said that herring is a unique animal: in fact, no other animals in the world are known to communicate with farts.

Manatees, Marine Animals That Swim Thanks to Their Farts

Much scientific evidence has now proved without fear of contradiction that the flatulence of manatees is the mechanism that helps them to swim. Manatees (Trichechus Linnaeus) are aquatic mammals that can reach three meters in length and weigh over 500 kilograms. They live in the waters of America, Africa and the Caribbean Sea. Scholars have become fond of these curious animals, which seem to have given rise to the legend of the mermaids.

The strangest thing is that these animals, considered as intelligent as dolphins, do not have a swim bladder. This organ is present in fish and helps them float, sink to the depths or rise to the surface. How do manatees do such things if they don't have it? Simple: they emit flatulence that helps them deflate. If, on the other hand, they hold back the farts, they swell.

The flatulence of manatees: the art of farting

Manatees are completely vegetarian and feed on algae and other marine plants. They then accumulate a nice amount of intestinal gas which helps them move up and down. Unfortunately, even this perfect mechanism can get jammed. In fact, the researchers found that constipated manatees have a hard time orienting and moving. The solution? A nice laxative and everything go back to normal.

In December 2020, a satirical artist even dedicated a cartoon on his Instagram profile to the flatulence of manatees. In the image you can see a couple: he is in the water and she, eating an ice cream, is floating up. He tells her "Justine, come down! Stop eating that ice cream, you know you're lactose intolerant!" And she replies "NEVER! This is my life now!" Many thought it was a joke: but manatees really swim... to the sound of farts.

Having gas is a completely natural manifestation

Flatulence is typical of mammals, in reality almost all other animals emit it. It can be formed from simple air swallowed while eating or from gases produced by yeasts and bacteria that live in the intestine. Science tells us that the human being releases an average of 0.5 to 1.5 liters of gas per day, divided into a variable quantity between 10 and over 20 farts.

In short, as much as one can voluntarily control one's emissions, gas is produced inside the human body and must necessarily come out of it. Since it is an inevitable fact, let's at least try to get it out in a private moment and not in class (or worse at the table), risking to stun fellow farters and teachers. How about?

FART History

Cold-blooded animals (such as snakes) also emit flatulence. The sound of their fart is not comparable to that of humans, but the stench can be the same. Or worse!

A curiosity: according to some, the popular term "fart" derives from the action of undoing the "strap" (an ancient name for the belt of trousers), which was performed after dinner. According to others, it derives from the sharp noise caused by a leather belt being snapped.

Mo-China: Spit, Burps and Farts

Here I am at the fateful topic that I did not want to address, but alas it is becoming a problem in the family. In China it is customary to spit on the ground in any place, so much so that one finds spittoons everywhere and above all by the elevator, because it is normal to spit before taking the elevator, spit at the restaurant, spit at the supermarket, in a taxi or car out of the window, on a moped, while you are walking and you must be lucky that the wind does not blow your way. Then there is the free burp: you find yourself talking to someone and while he speaks the burps come out along with the words and you are not in the restaurant but in the office. It happened to me with a Chinese boy yesterday who is in charge of the translations of the drawings, if then you're at your own dining table is the norm. Finally, the real farts which fortunately are now limited compared to a time, but still free. For the Chinese it is good that these things come out of the body because it is the evil that we have inside, but I cannot bear that my otherwise educated children are now getting used to this and it becomes normal at the table. And now what do I do I let myself go to decay ... Do I let the evil come out of me? Hamlet question, the fact is that I just can't yet, and I feel more and more like Mulan who, trying to spit to show that she is a man, spits on herself because she is not able ...

10 things to know before going to China

Before going to China for work, study, vacation or for any other reason, there are ten things you need to know to be psychologically ready to face this country:

1. The taxi drivers do not speak English and hardly know any addresses: so before taking a taxi in China, have the address in Chinese and maybe even directions or street names that are near the place where you need to go. Don't even try to hope that a Chinese taxi driver knows what Hilton or Canton Fair is because any foreign or English name in Chinese changes completely. While in Italian the Hilton remains Hilton in Chinese it becomes something completely different. So before getting into a taxi, be prepared.

2. The camel syndrome: the Chinese, when they have to spit, spit. But before they spit, they pick up the phlegm and emit a guttural sound that hasn't reached the Western world. So to the ears of the newcomer to China it will seem that the person who is about to spit is about to have a syncope and is about to fall to the ground. Instead, he is just collecting in phlegm that he will spit on the ground shortly thereafter.

3. Toilets are for many but not for everyone: for some reason the Chinese are not convinced that they have to take their children to public toilets or in the restrooms of restaurants or shopping centers. Instead, they prefer that their children do their business in the open air, in nature, perhaps mindful of a bucolic China that no longer exists. Therefore, a bush or a hedge will always be more attractive than a public bathroom. Even a garbage can will have an excellent function as a toilet rather than a public bathroom. So, expect to see Chinese children relieving themselves everywhere.

4. The Turkish or the Chinese? The bathroom defined in Italian as "alla turca" is the classic bathroom used by all Chinese in all homes, restaurants, shopping centers, airports. So, from today on I will no longer call it Turkish, but Chinese! If you are not a fan of the squat toilet, then look for the disabled bathroom where the toilet is usually located. Only in Western restaurants and upscale shopping malls are there bathrooms with toilets. Yet more than once I entered these bathrooms with the toilet and found the marks of the shoes on the donut of the toilet, a sign that even there the Chinese have not resisted the position of the Turkish who, by now, is spontaneous to them.

5. Free burp: the open mouth burp complete with sound effects is considered normal in China; indeed, the Chinese believe that it is good for health to release this air that comes from the stomach. Instead, they are adamant that it hurts to hold it back. So, get your ears ready for the concert of liberating burps which are not done only by country people, but by anyone living in China, whether bricklayers or teachers or students.

6. Push and keep quiet: in China no one asks for "permission" and no one apologizes when they have to make their way through a crowd of people to get out of the subway. No one apologizes for pushing someone else by mistake or stepping on someone's foot and, at the same time, the person who was pushed or stepped on their foot does not complain at all. Everyone is silent and meanwhile they push, pass in front, slip out of the subway with their elbows. So be ready to elbow and take thrusts without saying a word.

7. The style of Herod and Salome, or serving the head on a silver platter: in Chinese restaurants, even in the most renowned, it is customary to serve chicken and duck with their head on the plate. Even in supermarkets, when you want to buy chicken, you have to be careful because often the package is all inclusive, that is, it includes the head. The head is considered a

delicious and succulent part, just as my grandmother thought, who never discarded anything. And here I find the first affinity between the Venetians of the past and the Chinese: nothing is thrown away, everything is eaten! Who started eating crow's feet first? The Chinese or the Venetians? Certainly, my grandmother ate them, I've seen her do it more than once.

8. Nudism is fashionable: those who go to China must prepare to see many people half-naked, especially in southern China where it is hot, more so than in the Po valley. Men have a tendency to pull their shirts up to their necks, showing their powerful abs to anyone who passes by on the street. Women try to wear as few inches of fabric as possible, perhaps in order not to sweat or to avoid washing too many sweat-soaked clothes. So, get ready for the summer nudism show.

9. The traffic is not suitable for the faint of heart: so, if you have cardiovascular problems don't go to China because you could run out of steam. Or when taking a taxi, I highly recommend not looking at the road.

10. Collars and helmets do not exist: do not be frightened if you see dogs running in city traffic, nor if you see a moped with an adult and two children on board, all without helmets, going in the wrong direction on the highway in the evening. In China it is business as usual. Here people who have a dog usually take it for a walk without a leash and, without a leash, cross streets and walk in very busy areas, always with the dog beside or in front. As for the helmet, no one wears it, neither on a scooter, nor on a bicycle, nor when two, three, even four people travel together on the same scooter.

Country Travel Etiquette

Never say "cin cin" during a toast in Japan: it is vulgar. Do not leave chopsticks stuck inside the rice: it hurts. And in Buddhist countries, the heads of children are not stroked.

Beijing wants to establish etiquette courses for Chinese who go on holiday abroad (140 million in 2014), because - between bad habits such as spitting, pushing in the queue and letting unwanted morsels fall from the mouth onto the restaurant table - they create image problems for the second biggest world economy. But how do Italians across the border behave? There are 12.7 million (compared to 17 in 2007) who, even for a few days, go on vacation abroad. If we tend to be a little more polite than the Chinese, especially in the Far East, we often appear coarse and decidedly provincial.

Cin cin

The adventure of one of our entrepreneurs in Tokyo is emblematic. To seal the deal, he raised his glass and invited to toast with a “cheer”. The partners blanched: in Japanese that term is the most vulgar meaning of "penis". But it was only the latest in a series of mistakes. He exchanged business cards with one hand and pocketed them immediately: gestures that testify to little consideration. The "business card" (the first approach of a very shy people) must always be given and taken with two hands. Then it must be looked at and kept on the table until the end of the meeting.

The gentleman then entered his guest's house without taking off his shoes. He did not bow to his wife, but shook her hand tightly: two manifestations of arrogance. He then refused the ritual cup of tea, saying he preferred coffee: it is a welcome sign and, if you don't like it, just bring it to your lips. He interrupted the customer and raised his tone of voice during the negotiation, risking to "make him lose face."

In the East you should never scream or lose patience, especially if you need help. Confucian philosophy, the basis of Far East societies, does not foresee rejection. Aggression shows weakness. If you get upset because the deal doesn't close, you risk losing it. Our friend then noisily blew his nose at the table: vulgarity comparable to farting in public in Europe. You have to dab and, if you really can't resist, you have to go to the bathroom.

On the plate

Traveling in different cultures it is easy to make a mistake. At the table in China, if you are a guest, never refuse the food offered. Just taste it. And you don't have to finish everything on your plate: you have to leave a few grains of rice to show that the meal was plentiful. And never plant chopsticks in a bowl of rice: it is a funeral practice.

In the Islamic world, on the other hand, crossing the legs showing the soles of shoes is an insult and can provoke violent reactions. At the end of the meal, the cup of coffee is constantly refilled. If you don't want any more, you don't have to cover it with your hand (offensive) but turn it over. And a woman must never touch a man in public: in Iran it is a crime. In the Middle East as in India, if you become friends with a person of the same sex, it is normal to walk hand in hand: it does not imply you are gay. Those who refuse deny friendship. And in the bazaars, you don't start bargaining if you don't want to buy a product: it's a job, not a game.

With joined hands

In India and in Buddhist countries it is unfortunate to caress the head of children, because it is the seat of the Sahasrara chakra: if touched by a stranger - perhaps impure - it must be healed as soon as possible with purification rites. Furthermore, women must not show their shoulders: an erogenous part as opposed to the belly, which is shown here naked from under the breasts to the pubis. Furthermore, never declare yourself an atheist: being European is equivalent to being Christian. The right answer, therefore, is "God is one".

People greet each other with joined hands, as if in prayer, not shaking hands. We must not touch the Brahmins, the priestly caste. And never touch people with your left hand: it is used for intimate hygiene. You eat with the right hand. A belch after lunch shows satisfaction. If you find yourself at dinner with a Sikh family, you must finish everything on your plate: leaving it behind is an insult to poverty.

In Australia, if you talk to an Aboriginal, you can touch him but do not look him in the eye: direct gaze violates their interiority. In Anglo-Saxon countries, the gesture we make in Italy with our fingers to order two beers at the bar is the most trivial offense.

The examples can go on. It is a jungle of deeds and words in which it is difficult to extricate oneself.

It Floats into Space

Several years ago, Prof. Gianfranco Miglio political scientist, jurist and great supporter of federalism was, so to speak, the ideologue of the Northern League to whom he attributed the mission of finally achieving federalism in Italy. The paths of the Como intellectual and of the league, however, became divergent to the point of conflict. The expression that a gentleman of the caliber of Hon. Umberto Bossi, using his legendary verbal elegance, used to express his thoughts on Prof. Miglio: 'a fart in space'. Just on the sidelines, but only to underline who we are dealing with, the league try to pass off the federalist reform as inspired by the thoughts of Prof. Miglio on which they have spent words of appreciation. Gentlemen! There is nothing to say.

The refined expression of the 'senatur' immediately came back to my memory as appropriate when I read of the request made by Minister Zaja : RAI to make fiction in dialect. Famous for the milk quota issue, the Venetian statesman argues that RAI 3 is an ideological channel. Maybe he would like it Network 4 style. the statesmen of the Po Valley, in addition to the identity of polenta taragna, support the policy of a shop oriented towards closure, discrimination and intolerance.

Deadly Flatulence, Or How to Fart in Space Without Risk

For astronauts, going to the bathroom has a completely different meaning from ours.

In a gravity-free environment, flatulence, which contains flammable gases, such as hydrogen, could be dangerous as well as polluting the environment.

Of course, in the absence of air, one cannot hope for a breath of air to take it away.

But China has found a clever solution. While the system adopted so far was based on a system similar to the one we know, but equipped with an air pump that practically sucked everything, according to Li Tanqiu, an aerospace expert, astronauts can be deprived of their intestinal gases easily.

On the Shenzhou-6 spacecraft, launched on October 15, 2005 in China, Chinese scientists have installed a new, very simple and effective toilet. On board the shuttle, the toilet was equipped with a soft plastic hose and a pumping device that practically placed inside the anus, relentlessly sucks feces and gas into a fixed container. In this way, uncontrolled emissions of gases are avoided and they are isolated in the container.

The one-day mission featured astronaut Yang Liwei.

Of course, this system should be suitable for anyone, or for those who are constipated or diarrheal, then eliminates cleaning problems and, for those who are listless, also avoids the burden of "squeezing"!

Orpheus Sang Burping: Henry Purcell and His Merry Companions

Gherardo delle Notte, the joyful violinist

Bonjour mesdames et messieurs, and welcome to a new appointment with L'Esprit de Finesse, the cultural review dedicated to the works that have made the history of elegance and good taste on this marble of God that is our planet. Today, at the request of the Lega delle Caste Fanciulle in favor of the Differentiated Collection, we will present some extracts from a poetic-musical masterpiece which, if it has not yet found the space it deserves in general culture, is certainly due to a plot hatched by strong powers.

Come on, let's get started.

Leaving out the twentieth century, about which my ignorance forces me to remain silent, I am firmly convinced that no other moment in the history of Western music has known a ferment equal to that which exploded in England in the forty years that separate 1660 from 1700. That era, in an attempt to rejuvenate a national musical idiom perceived as antiquated and brainy, the English king Charles II and his successors are very open to welcoming and supporting any musician who knows how to teach something new to their subjects. It is like the kick-off of an exciting marathon which, in those decades, saw composers from all over Europe rush to London.

At court, the young and breezy violinist Thomas Baltzar amazes the audience with the bizarre virtuosity typical of the German school, while a temperamental Neapolitan named Nicola Matteis makes "his violin speak as if it had a human voice". Pelham Humfre, a young boy trained as a singer at Chapel Royal, returns from a trip to Paris with great haughtiness, but also with the ability to compose the most poignant church music of his time.

At the theater, the now forgotten Thomas Morgan and Thomas Tollett adorn the hottest pieces with dances that would not be out of place at a Dublin fair, while the Moravian Gottfried Finger juggles with a French style full of clichés (which, however, he abandons in favor of a markedly Italian vein in his gaudy sonatas). Having made his way through the courtiers playing the flute - in every possible sense of the expression, if we are to believe the insinuations of the gossipy Earl of Rochester - the gracious Frenchman Jacques Paisible enchants audiences with wonderful overtures, while the Catalan Luis Grabu gives to the English their first fully sung theatrical play, in the style learned in France by the court composer Jean-Baptiste Lully. Everything is fresh, everything is new, everything is beautiful.

It is around the turn of the century that in London, in the workshop of the printer John Walsh, an amazing collection, object of the interest of this article, sees the light: The Catch Club, or, Merry Companions - La Società delle Catch. What is a catch? Anyone who has some smattering of music theory will understand me when I say "something like a canon", but let me try to explain it also to those who are fasting the discipline. This is a catch:

No instruments, just voices - in this case three. A first voice begins to intone a text on a full meaning melody, which in this case covers the lines "Under this stone lies Gabriel John, in the year of our Lord one thousand and one". At the end of this exposition, a second voice enters which repeats exactly the same melody just ended by the first, with the same words; in the meantime, the first voice goes on intoning a sequel to the first text on another melody, which fits with perfect harmony on the notes of the second voice: in this case, it is the one that covers the words "Cover his head with turf or stone, ' tis all one,' tis all one, with turf or stone ' tis all one ".

Once this second step is finished, a third voice enters and does the same thing: it starts intoning the melody and the text of the first voice from the beginning, while the one that was our first voice moves on to the third section of the music and the text: "Pray for the soul of gentle John, if you please you may, or let it alone: ' tis all one".

To put it briefly, it is as if the three voices were chasing each other trying to catch each other: from this derives the name of catch, which in English means, precisely, "to grab". It sounds cumbersome, but I hope that listening to the example will make it clearer. If you have not understood, do not worry: we will not dwell much on musical issues in the rest of the article.

Now, even if I have chosen a particularly slow and gloomy catch for my example, this musical form usually has other preferences. In fact, it was not born as something committed, but as an expedient to be provided to music amateurs to have fun singing together: although its use in public contexts (such as theatrical performances - is documented, the favorite places for the execution of a wrestling match are the house, the living room or the tavern. If, however, you think that only the same amateurs to whom they were intended dedicated themselves to the composition of such small things, you are very mistaken: to enclose a large part of the history of English music of the late 1600s in a small book it would be enough to intertwine the biographical events of the composers who contributed to the collection of the printer Walsh. First of all, for art and fame, is Henry Purcell.

I am not saying that it is possible to make a qualitative ranking of all composers who have ever lived; I'm just saying, if it were possible, Henry Purcell would be in the top five. It is a drastic statement, but I would be prepared to fight with any child under ten who shows willingness to prove me wrong.

Dead at the age of 36 from pneumonia (apparently, his careless lady had left him locked out on a cold autumn night) this genius used his short life to completely revolutionize his beloved England's music scene: the perfect mastery of three musical styles (Italian, English and French) rightly earned him the epithet of Orpheus Britannicus with which his fellow composers began to call him after his death. It is with this great name that we wish to open our résumé, immediately presenting the first gem born from his immortal pen and included by Walsh within his refined Catch Club.

Ah, the rustling of the branches! Ah, the murmuring of the streams! The text of this bonbon of elegance, of a very clear bucolic-pastoral mold, consists of the following dialogue between at least two characters, whom we will call A and B:

A: " Pox on you!"

B: "For a fop, your stomachs too queasy.

Cannot I belch and fart, your coxcomb, to ease me?

What if I let fly in your face, and shall please ye?"

A: " Fogh, fogh, how sour he smells, now he's at it again;

Out ye beast, I never met so nasty a man.

I'm not able to bear it".

B: "What the Devil d'ye mean?

No less than a Caesar decree'd with great reason,

No restraint should be laid on the bum or the weason,

For belching and farting were always in season".

The normal exchange of words between a weak-stomached fop and an inveterate fart gives the author the right hand for a musical picture whose apparently simple melody is constructed with great ingenuity; the initial pauses allow the insertion of some belches, prescribed by the original score.

Jean Honoré Fragonard, The swing, 1767

After this first taste, some of our readers may begin to make a false impression of our collection. They might even - Heaven forfend! - come to think that here we are talking about something immoral. I am offended. Numi, what an offense. What a shame. Come here Ambrose, get slapped.

There is nothing more wrong, as evidenced by the text of a clearly devotional catch, which covers a very famous episode of the Bible with a sublime poem. In it, the young and handsome widow Judith manages to save her city from a siege by seducing the leader of the enemy army, the Assyrian Holofernes, and then cutting off his head during the night. All the drama, all the pathos of such an affair of love and death is thus summarized by the Merry Companions, in a piece of rare poetry of which unfortunately there are no recordings:

When Judith had laid Holofernes in bed,

She pull'd out his falchion, and cut off his head;

The reason is plain: he'd have made her his whore,

So, she cut off his head as I told you before.

Ah, the betrayed leader! Ah, the deceptive whispers of the widow! Neither Caravaggio nor Gentileschi were able to illustrate the famous tale with equally happy brushstrokes! And yet with the author of this masterpiece, the organist Michael Wise of Salisbury Cathedral, the fate was not tender: repeatedly reproached by his superiors for annoying drunkenness, he ended up with the brain crushed by a blow of the sword for having had the unfortunate idea of insulting a night watchman.

Another theme dear to the world of the Catch Club is that of the relationships between the sexes. A pure and idealized love is the background to the entire collection, in which shy young and angelic youths wink languidly at their unrequited affections. One of the highest singers of such a sentiment was the great Purcell who, betraying a knowledge of the ancient Tuscan stil novo, tells of his tormented relationship with his beloved woman, a haughty girl named Giulia. Please note how the music marries the lyrics in this triumph of British sophistication.

Ah, the loving sighs! Ah, the sweetest - THE sweetest pains! For those not lucky enough to be able to enjoy the text in its original language, here is a quick translation:

Once, twice, thrice I Julia try'd:

The scornful puss as oft deny'd,

And since I can no better thrive,

I'll cringe to ne'er a bitch alive;

So, kiss my ass, disdainful sow,

Good claret is my mistress now.

Note also a further refinement in the musical rendering of the text when, at the entrance of the third voice, the pauses in the melody cause the listener to intertwine the first voice with the third; the result is that the two singers seem to say -"so kiss my ass - once, kiss my ass - twice, kiss my ass - three times ". Ah, great Francesco Petrarca! Even in England you are remembered!

The last piece we take into question for this succinct, albeit incomplete, analysis was born from the pen of another great and forgotten composer. Born in 1668, John Eccles belonged to a generation of musicians following Purcell's; a renewed interest in him has given us in recent years some recordings of his plays, evidence of an ingenious and captivating style which, in his day, was able to appeal to the fickle English public.

Its presence in the Merry Companions group is well demonstrated by one of the most famous pieces of the entire collection, expertly built around a very simple text that has made generations of scholars sweat. It is the same score that illustrates, in a short introduction, the trivial episode that is the background to the wonderful verses with which it has been covered: "Mary, my maid, one day broke the handle of her brush, and when she learned that my servant John had a stick that could have replaced it, he asked him to put it in the brush for her.' What the anonymous poet - perhaps the composer himself? - managed to draw from this minutia is a delightful and polite portrait of domestic intimacy:

Jean Honoré Fragonard, The Blind Hen, 1750

My man John had a thing that was long,

My maid Mary had a thing that was hairy;

My man John put his thing that was long

Into my maid Mary's thing that was hairy.

My maid Mary then stirr'd it about,

Till with stirring and stirring at length it came out,

But then my man John thrust it in once again,

And knock'd it most stoutly to make it remain.

But John with much knocking so widen'd the hole,

That his long thing slip'd out still in spight of his soul;

Till weary'd and vex'd and with knocking grown sore,

Cry'd: "A pox take the hole, for I'll knock it no more!"

Numerous hypotheses have been advanced on the interpretation of this poetic miniature. What on earth will hide behind the author's daring metaphors? Do the names of John and Mary refer to the eternal mystery that surrounds the figure of the apostle John in Leonardo da Vinci's Last Supper, identified by some as Mary Magdalene? Does the hole mentioned in the last quatrain have some connection with Horace's immortal couplet "My Father, if I don't get married - I'll die without that thing"? Could the "long thing" of the servant John refer to the swords of the Knights Templar, who defended the city of Acre from the siege of the Saracens in 1291? We may never know.

Many other wonders are hidden within this collection, which only the editorial needs prevent me from delving deeper. Those readers who enjoy music can easily find a complete scan on the net, and I assure you from direct experience that an evening with friends with wine and catch can be a fantastic remedy for the tensions accumulated during a working day.

Thank you for joining us in this new appointment with L'Esprit de Finesse, the beacon of good taste in an Internet made up of sex, filth and “rather than” used with a disjunctive function.

Why Do the Jackets... Stink?

In this chapter we talk about farts. Okay, don't make that face because all mammals do. Find out what the origin is

Or, if you prefer the scientific term, flatulence. That is, as the dictionary says, of the noisy emission of intestinal gas from the anus.

Have you ever found yourself in a closed place, for example an elevator, and smelt a devastating smell, with other people there with you turning from side to side, pretending nothing or looking at the time?

Worse still if someone comes out of the elevator or some other small enclosed place and has decided to leave a gift just for you as you enter.

In fact, apart from the hilarity and disgust they cause in public, we all do fart in private. But everyone! Males, females, cats, dogs.

I know it's not poetic to imagine the girl you're in love with farting. But fate is cynical and cheating: she makes them too; this is the truth. Rihanna and Rita Ora, Lionel Messi and Cristiano Ronaldo, Lebron James and Stephen Curry also make them.

You will say: yes, oh well, once or twice it happens. No no, my dear. Between burps (precisely belching) and farts (precisely flatulence) humans eliminate excess gases (carbon dioxide, oxygen, nitrogen, hydrogen and sometimes methane) by doing 14-15 farts a day, enough to eliminate, on average, from 0.5 liters to two liters

THE CAUSE

The terrible stench of fart is caused by bacteria that release sulfur-containing gases in the intestine. The gas comes from the ingestion of air and bacteria present in the large intestine (colon). We all ingest small amounts of air when we eat and drink. But if we eat and drink quickly, if we are in the habit of chewing gum, smoking or having dental implants, we ingest more air.

The same air can take the elevator and go up or down. Upward it goes faster and that's why we burp more on average than we fart. When we do not digest food, it goes from the small to the large intestine, where the bacterial flora digests a part of it producing hydrogen, carbon dioxide and, in many people but not all, methane: these gases are expelled from the floor below...

BUT WHAT FOODS ... PRODUCE GAS?

Attention, battalion! If you want to do a few gases, you don't have to eat these things a lot! But if you don't mind a lot of gas, you can eat these delicacies! Watch out, go!

Oh, my goodness, it's hard to find foods that don't produce gas. Think about how many there are that contain carbohydrates, gather in meditation and sum up, because they can cause the formation of gas.

Your beloved sugars, dear gluttons, are no less. Among these, raffinose, lactose, fructose and sorbitol produce gas. And where are they located? Hear hear: raffinose is in beans, asparagus, broccoli, cabbage, whole grains and various vegetables. Lactose is in milk, cheese, bread, your beloved ice cream, salads, cereals, dressings. Fructose is in pears, artichokes, onions, wheat, some sodas and some fruit juices. Sorbitol is in peaches, apples, pears and prunes, sweeteners and diet foods, candy and chewing gum.

Starches - such as those in pasta, wheat and potatoes - produce gas, while rice produces no gas. So, you ask yourself, the Chinese who eat a lot of rice, don't they fart? I wouldn't say it, especially if they put seasonings in the rice. But let's go ahead and try to end the list here, which takes me despondent.

Soluble and insoluble fiber is found in beans, peas, oat bran, and most fruit. So, in conclusion, I can only tell you this: either eat other things, if you find them, or save those who can ...

Longest Fart Ever? Ray Broom's, With 2 Minutes And 47 Seconds

The longest and most unbeatable fart

The longest fart ever released in history dates back to several years ago and still no person has managed to do better. The chronometer spoke clearly, even if it was not easy to formalize the record. In fact, one can only imagine the bad smell caused by this infinite flatulence. The 167 seconds overall attracted an infinite number of very fierce challengers. World Fart Day is the right time to try to overtake Ray Broom.

World Days are a fairly recent innovation. One of the most memorable ones is undoubtedly dedicated to farts. There is no need to be ashamed of anything in this society, not even the longest fart ever emitted on this planet. The singular primacy was conquered some time ago by a certain Ray

Broom (the surname seems almost an onomatopoeic description of his flatulence).

No one has ever managed to do better than his 2 minutes and 47 seconds, a truly infinite time if you think about what it refers to. How the hell did he do it? Oddly, there is great mystery on the net about Broom's world record. His longest fart - when was it done? You can imagine the "judges" in charge of timing the time with gas masks and all possible precautions.

Very little information

There are also no images and the official Guinness World Record website makes no reference to this area, focusing instead on the burps. How then do you say that the man is the bizarre record holder? In online forums, nothing else is talked about and Broom is constantly cited by his bitter and fierce opponents.

In fact, on the occasion of every world day dedicated to intestinal gas (September 20 to be precise), the challenge is launched and many people say they are sure they can do better than the longest fart ever. Those 167 seconds have been resisting since time immemorial, even tricks such as heavy dishes and propitiatory ingredients (beans in the first place, as you can imagine) were not enough to conquer the coveted and smelly crown.

www.ingramcontent.com/pod-product-compliance
Lightning Source LLC
Chambersburg PA
CBHW051025030426
42336CB00015B/2717
* 9 7 8 1 7 7 7 0 1 1 4 9 9 *